examination
of the urine
Second Edition

examination
of the urine
Second Edition

A PROGRAMMED TEXT

John M. Weller, M.D.
Director, Nephrology Service,
University Hospital,
The University of Michigan;
Professor of Internal Medicine,
The University of Michigan,
Ann Arbor, Michigan

and

James A. Greene III, M.D.
Director, Michigan Nephrology Center,
Kalamazoo, Michigan;
Associate Clinical Professor,
College of Human Medicine,
Michigan State University,
East Lansing, Michigan

APPLETON-CENTURY-CROFTS/New York

Library of Congress Cataloging in Publication Data

Weller, John M
  Examination of the urine, a programmed text.

  1. Urine—Analysis and pathology—Programmed
instruction. I. Greene, James A., 1930-   joint
author. II. Title. [DNLM: 1. Urine—Analysis—Programmed texts. QY18 W448e]
RB53.W44 1976   616.07'566'077   76-12721
ISBN 0-8385-2319-6

Prentice-Hall International, Inc., London
Prentice-Hall of Australia, Pty. Ltd., Sydney
Prentice-Hall of India Private Limited, New Delhi
Prentice-Hall of Japan, Inc., Tokyo
Prentice-Hall of Southeast Asia (Pte.) Ltd., Singapore

PRINTED IN THE UNITED STATES OF AMERICA

Cover design: The Old Typosopher

The authors wish to express their appreciation to George L. Geis, Ph.D., Center for Research on Learning and Teaching, The University of Michigan, for assistance in the preparation of this teaching program and to Paul Borondy for the photomicrographs of urine sediments.

The preparation of this programmed material was supported in part by a grant from the National Fund for Medical Education.

With the permission of The Williams & Wilkins Company, Dr. Weller has used portions of his chapter, "The Urinary System," from their 8th edition of Miller and Weller: *Textbook of Clinical Pathology* (1971).

introduction

Examination of the urine is the most frequently utilized of all clinical laboratory tests, and it is the simplest. It is useful in disclosing disease or disturbed function of the kidneys, ureters, bladder, or urethra. It also aids in ascertaining the presence of certain systemic diseases that cause abnormalities in the urine. Examination of the urine is the most important laboratory procedure done in the initial evaluation of the patient.

It is the purpose of this presentation to enable the student to examine the urine properly and to interpret correctly the results of the various tests that are usually carried out on the urine. These tests are of certain physical aspects (volume, appearance, color and specific gravity or osmolality) and of various chemical constituents (hydrogen ion, protein, hemoglobin, sugar, ketones, phenylpyruvic acid and bilirubin), as well as for identification of the formed elements (red blood cells, white cells, epithelial cells, casts, and crystals) and determining presence or absence of bacteriuria. Details of these tests are given in Part 2, "Methods for Examination of the Urine." It is not intended that the student will memorize these; he should refer to them as they are needed.

Any laboratory procedure must be carried out properly to provide a meaningful result. In interpreting the result one must draw on knowledge of both normal structure and function of the human body and of alterations produced by disease. A well-trained technician can perform laboratory tests accurately. The physician, however, bears the responsibility for correctly interpreting the results of such tests. He must utilize his knowledge of the laboratory procedure itself, the deviations from normal resulting from disease, and the clinical state of his patient. This instructional material is designed to assist the medical student in developing the facility to correlate these items of information, so that when presented with abnormal findings derived from examining the urine, he will know what pathophysiologic processes can be responsible.

Learning to recognize the formed elements seen on microscopic examination of the urinary sediment is particularly difficult. Words usually fail to convey adequate descriptions, so that it is necessary for the student to gain this ability to recognize through repeated observations. This requires considerable time. An integral part of the programmed instructional material presented here is the provision of black-and-white and color photographs that are utilized in conjunction with the text. By this means the student can learn readily to identify the formed elements commonly seen in the urinary sediment.

The photomicrographs of the formed elements found in the urinary sediment are of actual urine sediments derived from patients seen in the clinic. A tabulation of the formed elements shown in these black-and-white and color photographs of the urine sediments is presented in Part 3, "Atlas of Urine Sediments."

This programmed text has undergone repeated evaluations and revisions. Not only has its use permitted a reduction in time allotted for the presentation and study of this subject, but it has also resulted in increased effectiveness of instruction (J Med Educ 42:697, 1967).

This instructional material is designed for use in a clinical laboratory diagnosis course in medical school. That its usefulness is not confined to this group of students has become apparent as others have sought it out. Medical technologists, residents in internal medicine, residents in clinical pathology, and practicing physicians have all found it to be of value. It is offered, therefore, to all who wish to learn how to examine the urine, either for the first time or for recall and revitalization of an old acquaintanceship.

contents

PART 1. PROGRAMMED INSTRUCTIONAL MATERIAL ON EXAMINATION OF THE URINE

PART 2. METHODS FOR EXAMINATION OF THE URINE

instructions to the student

This material on examination of the urine is presented in the form of a self-instructional program, so that the student may set his own pace for achieving the stated goals. It is arranged in three sections. Do not attempt to master all sections of the program at one sitting. If too much time has elapsed between working on a section, a short review will be beneficial.

Write your answers in the spaces provided. Actually writing the answer is most important. When choices are given in parentheses, circle the correct answer. Confirm that your written answer is correct by turning the page and looking at the identically numbered item in the left-hand (answer) box. *Give yourself credit for being right if you have put down a synonym for the correct answer.* A few synonyms are given in parentheses. If your answer is *wrong, reread* the item and determine how to arrive at the correct response. Pay attention and think actively. Do not cheat yourself by looking at the answer on the next page before you write it down in the space provided.

Each numbered paragraph of the programmed material is termed a "frame." Occasionally you will be referred to frames on other pages of the program. The black-and-white pictures are given consecutive figure numbers (eg, Figure 1) and will be found in Part 3; pages 149-60. The color photomicrographs are also numbered consecutively. They will be found in Part 3, pages 161-68. Look carefully at the black-and-white and color figures when you are asked to do so.

Starting at the top of page 1, fill in frame 1. Then turn to page 3 and look at the answer in the left-hand box at the top of the page. The answer to frame 1 is also number 1. If your answer is wrong, reread frame 1 and correct your answer. If your initial answer is correct, continue on to frame 2, the right-hand box at the top of page 3. Its answer will be found in the left-hand box at the top of page 5. Follow along in this fashion through the entire program. When you finish you will know how to examine the urine.

examination
of the urine
Second Edition

PART 1

programmed
instructional material
on examination
of the urine

Collection of Urine Specimens

Urine must be collected so that it is not contaminated by material from outside the urinary tract, such as in the female by vaginal material, or that from dirty containers, because the presence of contaminants may lead to _____ interpretation of the urine examination.

(Now turn to page 3 and stay in the top strip.)

Turn to page 3, answer frame 1.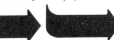

1

---

hematuria

Hemoglobin in the urine is called _____ and can be identified by chemical test.

64

65

---

contamination
with foreign
material

inadequately re-
suspended sample

failure to use both
low and high
magnifications

use of too much
light

drying of the sedi-
ment

128

The results of examination of a urine sediment that is prepared from a 12 ml aliquot of urine, centrifuged at 1500 rpm for five minutes, resuspended in 0.5 ml of urine, placed on a slide, and covered with a cover slip (are) (are not) identical with a urine sediment prepared from the same volume of urine which is not centrifuged.

(Circle the correct answer.)

129

squamous epithelial cells	These cells obviously do not arise from the urinary tract. This specimen was most likely collected from a (male) (female) patient. Why? Because the urine was contaminated with _____ . (Circle the correct answer.)
192	**193**

A. Red blood B. Fine granular	By its size one would classify **B** as a _____ cast.
256	**257**

A. Oval fat body B. Red blood cell C. fragment of red blood cell cast D. Hyaline cast *(If you missed* **A**, *review frames 272 to 282.)*	On color Figure 39 on page 168, high power, stained, name the following: *Just below* **A.** _____ . **B.** A degenerating renal tubular epithelial cell cast containing coarse granules and _____ . *End of line* **C.** _____ .
320	**321**

wrong
(faulty)

Urine specimens from females may contain contaminants such as squamous epithelial cells and
other_____leading to
wrong_____.

1 | 2

---

hemoglobinuria

Many red cells or much hemoglobin in the urine
will color it _____ or _____.

65 | 66

---

are not

The difference in these urine sediments is in the
_____of formed elements.

129 | 130

female

vaginal material

193

In color Figure 9 on page 162, high power, stained, look closely at the nuclei and identify the follow- ing cells:

A. _____.
B. _____.

194

---

broad

257

Identify the following elements in the stained sediment shown in high-power color Figure 24, page 165:

A. _____.
B. *(the cast)* _____.
C. _____.
D. _____.

258

A. Red blood cell
B. Fat droplets
C. Red blood cell

321

Look at the nucleus of the cell at the end of the line from **D** on color Figure 39. It is (lobulated) (not lobulated). This cell is a _____.

322

vaginal material interpretation	Urine collected in a poorly washed bedpan that has previously been used by a patient given mineral oil may contain oil droplets. If the bedpan has been wiped with a towel, fibers may be found in the urine. (Look at Figure 1 in Part 3 on page 149.) In Figure 1, a low-power magnification, the contaminants are (oil droplets) (fibers) (vaginal material).
	(Circle the correct answer.)
2	**3**

red brown	Excessive intravascular hemolysis, such as occurs with a transfusion reaction or after ingestion of naphthalene moth balls, results in red or brown urine because of the presence of (red blood cells) (hemoglobin).
	(Circle the correct answer.)
66	**67**

concentration (number)	Sometimes the formed elements in the urine are so numerous that they are seen to better advantage when the urine is not concentrated by _____ .
130	**131**

A. Poly (Stern-heimer-Malbin positive) **B.** Renal tubular epithelial cell	In color Figure 9 the most common cell is a _____ cell.
194	**195**
A. Red blood cell **B.** Coarse granu-lar cast **C.** Red blood cell **D.** Red blood cell	The granules in cast **B** are not as coarse as in some casts. As a cellular cast degenerates, the cast first appears as a _____ cast and then as a _____ cast.
258	**259**
(lobulated) normal poly	Figure 22, on page 159, low power, stained, is a _____.
322	**323**

(fibers)

Urine need not be collected in a sterile container, but it must be collected in _____ containers.

3

4

(hemoglobin)

In determining whether the presence of red blood cells or that of hemoglobin is the cause of red or brown urine, one can identify red cells by _____ examination and detect hemoglobin by_____ test.

67

68

centrifugation

In order to make the results of the examination of the urine meaningful, the _____ of magnification used for counting the number of formed elements should be recorded.

131

132

renal tubular epithelial	Figure 7 on page 152 is a high-power view, stained, of a _____ cell.
195	**196**

coarse granular fine granular	It is rare, but the contents of a cast may become so homogenous that a waxy-appearing material forms, called a _____ cast.
259	**260**

fiber	The number of fibers and other extraneous materials will be kept at a minimum if the clean voided midstream urine sample is collected in a _____ container.
323	**324**

clean

The proteinaceous formed elements (red cells, white cells, and casts) may deteriorate if urine is not examined within four hours. Urine may be *preserved* to prevent deterioration of the _____ _____ .

4

5

microscopic

chemical

The presence of hematuria is verified _____ .

68

69

power

Therefore, when you record your results you indicate

A. whether the urine was or was not _____ , and

B. what _____ was used.

132

133

squamous epithelial	Figure 8 on page 152 is a *low-power* view of the unstained urine sediment from a female patient who had the classic symptoms of active urinary tract infection, ie, fever, flank pain, and dysuria. The small cells (**A**) are probably polys, and the very large cells (**B**) are _____ cells.
196	**197**
waxy	Unlike the hyaline cast, which is best seen with _____ illumination, the refractile homogenous waxy cast can be seen with or without _____ illumination.
260	**261**
clean	Identify the following on color Figure 40 on page 168, high power, stained: A. _____ . B. *(large)* _____ . C. _____ . *Cell at end of line* D. _____ .
324	**325**

formed elements	The formed elements (_____ _____) should be *preserved* by one of several ways if examination of the urine is delayed beyond _____.
5	6

microscopically	The presence of hemoglobinuria is verified _____.
69	70

A. centrifuged B. magnification (power)	In order to make the drop of urine sediment being examined more uniform in depth on the slide, it should always be covered with a _____ _____.
133	134

squamous epithelial **197**	Figure 9 on page 153 is a high-power view of the previous unstained urine sediment. What is the predominant cell? **198**
reduced reduced **261**	Since waxy casts tend to be found when renal failure occurs and the renal tubules are dilated, they are also usually _____ casts. **262**
A. Squamous epithelial cell B. Fat droplet C. Transitional epithelial cell D. Red blood cell *(If you missed C, go back to frames 184-187.)* **325**	In Figure 5, on page 151, unstained (note that this is low power), identify: *Object at very end of line* A. _____ _____ . *Objects at end of line* B. _____ _____ . **326**

red cells, white
cells, and casts

four hours

6

Urine should be examined within _____
because _____
_____ .

7

---

chemically

70

Of course, when there is either hematuria or hemoglobinuria, the chemical test for hemoglobin will be (positive) (negative).

(Circle the correct answer.)

71

---

cover slip

134

The results of repeated urine sediment examinations on a patient can be compared if they are collected over similar periods of time and are prepared from aliquots of urine having the same _____ and handled in the same way, ie, centrifuged for_____minutes at _____ rpm, and _____in 0.5 ml of urine, placed on a slide, and covered with a_____.

135

Poly	Notice in Figure 9 that many of these cells, like **A** and **B**, have relatively clear cytoplasm and appear (shrunken) (swollen).
	(Circle the correct answer.)
198	**199**

broad	In the center of the field of color Figure 25 on page 165 (lower end of unlabeled line) is shown a low-power view, unstained, of a _____ cast. **A** is a _____ cell.
262	**263**

A. Hyaline cast **B.** Oval fat bodies *(At this magnification you could not distinguish oval fat bodies from oil droplets.)*	Identify the labeled items in Figure 2 on page 149, high power, unstained. Look carefully at both ends of object **A**. Note that **B** and **C** look alike, although they are different sizes. **A.** _____ . **B.** _____ . **C.** _____ .
326	**327**

four hours

formed elements
may deteriorate

In this graph of bacterial growth, the increased
_____ of bacteria in unpreserved
contaminated urine may result in utilization of
any _____ present.

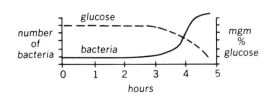

7

8

(positive)

Chemical tests for hemoglobin in the urine will be
positive in patients having either _____
or _____ .

71

72

---

volume

five

1500

resuspended

cover slip

Results are recorded as the number of casts per
_____ and the number of
cells per _____ .

135

136

(swollen)

199

This swelling of the cell is due to the urine's being _____, ie, having an osmolality _____ 310 mOsm/kg water.

200

broad waxy

squamous epithelial

263

Granular casts may contain hemoglobin pigment if they were originally _____ casts.

264

A. Fiber
B. Oil (fat droplet)
C. Oil (fat droplet)

327

Urine may be preserved by

A. _____ .
B. _____ .
C. _____ .

Check the best method for preservation of the formed elements. Put two checks in front of the method that is best for preservation of the urine for chemical examination.

328

number glucose	The metabolism of bacteria growing in urine will utilize any glucose present. A urine specimen for glucose analysis should be _____ if it is not to be tested within _____ hours.
8	**9**

hematuria hemoglobinuria	**Examination of the Urinary Sediment** Figure 2 on page 149 is a high-power view of a sediment from urine voided into a bedpan and transferred into a container that has been poorly rinsed. As you can see, the urinary sediment may contain elements, such as fibers and oil droplets, that were _____ present when the urine was in the bladder.
72	**73**

low-power field high-power field	Urine sediments can be satisfactorily compared if collected similarly and then handled in the same way—ie, the drop of urine sediment is covered with a _____ and the cells and casts are reported as number per _____ field.
136	**137**

hypotonic less than	In the high-power view shown in color Figure 6 on page 162, stained, identify: *below* B. _____ . C. _____ .
200	**201**
red blood cell	In color Figure 26 on page 166, high-power view, unstained, the group of cells at **A** constitute a _____ .
264	**265**

√√refrigeration
    at 4 C
 	
adding 2 ml
    toluene
 	
√ adding 8 drops
    10 percent
    formalin per
    30 ml urine
	Draw diagramatic crystals of
	
	A. calcium oxalate.
	
	B. triple phosphate.

328	**329**

preserved four	Bacterial growth, in addition to its utilization of _____ , may produce ammonia fròm urea. Ammonia combines with hydrogen ions to form ammonium ions. This alters the urine pH. The urine pH will_____ .
9	**10**
not	Figure 2 shows the presence of _____ and_____ .
73	**74**
cover slip high- or low-power	The staining characteristics of formed elements in the urine may aid in their identification. The sediment should be examined before and after being _____ .
137	**138**

below **B.** Transitional epithelial cell.

(If you missed **B,** *return to frame 184.)*

C. Poly (normal)

(If you called this a renal tubular epithelial cell, look at frame 180.)

201

Figure 10 on page 153 is an oil immersion view of an unstained group (**A**) of _____ . Under the microscope, Brownian motion of their cytoplasmic _____ could be seen.

202

red blood cell cast

265

Color Figure 27 on page 166 is a view under oil immersion, unstained. Identify:

A. _____ .
B. _____ .
C. _____ .
D. _____ .

266

A.

B.

329

Chemical Examination of the Urine

Determining the pH of urine may provide important clues about disease processes, acid-base balance, or functional ability of the renal tubule to excrete _____ ions.

pH is the negative log of the _____ concentration. We express the alkalinity or acidity of the urine in terms of _____ units.

330

glucose rise (increase)	Bacterial growth and metabolism after_____hours will alter the results of two chemical tests on the urine. These are tests for A. _____. B. _____.
10	**11**
a fiber oil droplets	Since urine is rarely collected in *sterile* containers, even urine that is sterile when voided and collected in a clean container may contain contaminants, such as _____, after it has stood long enough at room temperature.
74	**75**
stained	After the urine sediment has been resuspended, the Sternheimer-Malbin stain is done by adding two drops of _____ stain to 0.5 ml of urine. One drop of this mixture is placed on a slide and covered with a _____.
138	**139**

polys (WBCs) granules	If these polys in Figure 10 were Sternheimer-Malbin positive, the nuclei would stain _____ and the cytoplasmic granules would stain _____ .
202	**203**

A. Red blood cell B. Red blood cell C. Red blood cell D. Red blood cell cast	If you called this a granular cast you were wrong, because most of the cells in this cast can still be recognized as _____ cells.
266	**267**

hydrogen hydrogen ion pH	The pH of urine is usually measured clinically by the color of Nitrazine® paper after it has been dipped in the urine. As the renal tubule is the only mechanism that the body has for eliminating nonvolatile acids, the pH of urine is usually _____ .
330	**331**

four glucose pH **11**	If urine is not examined within four hours, elevation of the pH may be a factor causing formed elements to _____ . **12**
bacteria **75**	Two ways to avoid the confusion caused by bacterial proliferation are A. to examine the urine _____ ; or B. to _____ the growth of bacteria by some method of preservation. **76**
Sternheimer- Malbin cover slip **139**	The Sternheimer-Malbin stain stains nuclear elements of normal cells purple. Look at color Figure 1, on page 16, high power. There you will see the purple nucleus of a normal poly stained with the _____ stain. (Composition of this stain is given in Part 2, "Methods for Examination of the Urine," on pages 132-33.) **140**

pale blue slate gray **203**	In Figure 10 on page 153 name cell **B**. **204**
red blood **267**	Color Figure 28 on page 166, high power, unstained, shows a cast in which the cells are not identifiable. It should be called a _____ cast. **268**
low (acid) **331**	The metabolism of sulfur-containing amino acids of protein necessitates the loss of sulfate as well as _____ ions in the urine. **332**

deteriorate

Therefore, if chemical tests on, or microscopic examination of, the urine is not to be done within _____ hours, the urine should be _____ .

12

13

A. immediately
B. inhibit (pre-
   vent)

The bacterial growth curve below was seen when urine in a clean (nonsterile) container stood at room temperature. Urine should be examined before (two) (four) (six) hours.

(Circle the correct answer.)

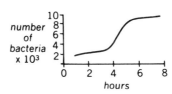

76

77

Sternheimer-
Malbin

The color of the nucleus of a normal poly stained with the Sternheimer-Malbin stain is _____ .

140

141

Red blood cell	Color Figure 10 on page 162 is an oil immersion view of a urine sediment stained with the Sternheimer-Malbin stain. Cell **A** is a _____ _____ .
204	**205**
coarse granular	This cast contains _____ pigment; it was most likely a _____ cast.
268	**269**
hydrogen	Urine pH ranges from a maximal acidity of 4.5 to a maximal alkalinity of 8.0 units. This is usually measured with _____ .
332	**333**

four

preserved

If unsterile urine is not examined within four hours, there may be _____ , and this may lead to

A. _____

B. _____

C. _____

13   **14**

(four)

Ideally, the urine sediment should be examined _____ but at least within _____ hours of voiding unless it is _____ .

77   **78**

---

purple

(Some may call this pink or red; others, orange. We will call it purple.)

The color of the nucleus of certain abnormal polys stained with the Sternheimer-Malbin stain is pale blue. These are called Sternheimer-Malbin positive cells. The blue color of their nuclei contrasts with the color of the nuclei of normal polys, which is _____ .

141   **142**

Sternheimer- Malbin positive poly	Cell **B** is a _____ .
205	**206**
hemoglobin red blood cell	The granules in the cast shown in color slide D29, high power, unstained, are (coarse) (fine).
269	**270**
Nitrazine® paper	The maximal acidity of the urine is about _____ pH units.
333	**334**

growth of bacteria present

ammonium formation with increase of pH

utilization of any glucose present

degeneration of formed elements

14

Urine voided on arising in the morning is normally more concentrated and therefore contains _____ formed elements per unit volume.

15

---

immediately

four

preserved

Most cells or casts found in urine contain protein as a major constituent. Protein tends to be less soluble in acid solutions and more soluble in _____ solutions.

78

79

---

purple

The Sternheimer-Malbin stain is most useful in identifying the Sternheimer-Malbin positive polys, which have nuclei that stain _____ in color. Sternheimer-Malbin positive polys are associated with urinary tract infection.

142

143

renal tubular epithelial cell	Color Figure 11 on page 163 is an oil immersion view, stained. Cell **A** is a _____.
206	**207**

fine	The color of this cast is due to _____ _____ indicating that it was a _____ .
270	**271**

4.5	Alkaline urine may be present in the following situations: **A.** After ingestion of sodium _____ _____ . **B.** After vomiting gastric contents containing _____ . **C.** When bacteria in the urine cause formation of _____ from urea.
334	**335**

more

Very dilute urine, being _____ tonic as compared to a protein-free filtrate of plasma (specific gravity 1.008), makes formed elements swell and be disrupted. Red cells will lyse in a _____ tonic fluid such as distilled water (specific gravity 1.000).

15

16

alkaline

Most formed elements in the urine sediment, such as red cells, white cells, and casts, have as a major constituent protein that is less soluble in acid solutions and more soluble in _____ solutions.

79

80

pale blue

Since the nucleus of the Sternheimer-Malbin positive poly stains blue, in contrast to the purple nuclei of normal polys, this stain is most useful in identifying the _____ poly.

143

144

Sternheimer-Malbin positive poly	In cell **A** on color Figure 11 we can tell that the urine is _____ tonic because the cytoplasm is _____ .
207	208

hemoglobin pigment red blood cell cast	In nephrotic renal disease, fat droplets accumulate in renal tubular epithelial cells and macrophages. In so-called oval fat bodies these _____ can be seen within the cell.
271	272

A. bicarbonate (or other buffer anion) B. hydrochloric acid C. ammonia	The pH of urine ranges from _____ to _____ units and is usually measured by using _____ _____ .
335	336

hypo hypo	Formed elements remain in a better state of preservation when the urine, compared to a protein-free filtrate of plasma, is _____ tonic or _____ tonic.
16	**17**
alkaline	Formed elements in alkaline solutions tend to (precipitate) (dissolve). (Circle the correct answer.)
80	**81**
Sternheimer- Malbin positive	Look at cell B in color Figure 2, on page 161, high power. The nucleus of this poly is stained pale blue. Such polymorphonuclear leukocytes, seen in association with urinary tract infections, having nuclei stained pale blue instead of purple, are called _____cells.
144	**145**

hypo swollen	Cell **B** on color Figure 11 is a _____ _____ cell, and the large, ill-defined cell in the far left-lower corner having a nucleus that is about the size of cell **B** is probably a _____ _____ cell.
208	209
fat droplets	Renal tubular epithelial cells, or phagocytic cells filled with fat droplets, are called oval _____ bodies.
272	273
4.5 8.0 Nitrazine® paper	Proteinuria occurs when increased glomerular permeability allows greater passage of plasma proteins. Protein in the urine is called _____ .
336	337

iso hyper 17	Urine voided on arising in the morning is better for microscopic examination because it is more _____. It therefore contains more _____ _____ . 18
(dissolve) 81	Therefore, the formed elements, _____ , _____ , and _____ , are more soluble in urine with an _____ pH and are (more) (less) readily seen on microscopic examination. (Circle the correct answer.) 82
Sternheimer- Malbin positive 145	The Sternheimer-Malbin stain, a mixture of safranin and crystal violet, stains the _____ of normal polys a _____ color. 146

renal tubular
epithelial

squamous
epithelial

Identify the following in color Figure 12 on page 163, high power, stained (look carefully at the cells in which the lines end):

A. _____ cell.
B. _____ .
C. _____ cell.
D. _____ .

209

210

---

fat

Fat droplets are highly refractile and somewhat brownish in color. When massed together, they appear as dark brown objects, so that cells filled with fat droplets can be identified by their darkness and brown color as _____ bodies.

273

274

---

proteinuria

Albumin, having a smaller molecular weight, passes through the _____ more easily than globulin; therefore, the protein in urine is mainly _____ .

337

338

concentrated (hypertonic)	These formed elements are not likely to lyse because the urine is *not* _____ tonic.
formed elements per unit volume	
18	**19**

red cells	If bacteria metabolize urea to form ammonia, the urine pH will (rise) (fall).
white cells	
casts	(Circle the correct answer.)
alkaline	
(less)	
82	**83**

nuclei	The Sternheimer-Malbin positive poly has a homogenous nucleus that is _____ in color and slate gray cytoplasmic granules. Look at cell **B** in color Figure 2, on page 161. The cell nucleus primarily takes up the crystal violet stain. The cytoplasmic granules are (purple) (slate gray).
purple	
	(Circle the correct answer.)
146	**147**

A. Squamous
    epithelial

*(If you missed
this, return to
frame 187.)*

B. Sternheimer-
    Malbin
    positive poly
C. Red blood
D. Sternheimer-
    Malbin
    positive poly

210

In color Figure 4 on page 161, high power, unstained, cell **A** has a nucleus even though it is out of the field. Cells **B** and **C** do not have nuclei.

Identify the following three cells:

A. _____ cell.
B. _____ cell.
C. _____ cell.

211

---

oval fat

274

In Figure 12 on page 154, unstained, low power, the highly refractile dark objects around cast **B** are

_____ .

275

---

glomerular
membrane
(glomerulus)

albumin

338

Determining the magnitude of albuminuria is of diagnostic importance, as in diseases causing the nephrotic syndrome there are usually more than 3.5 g albumin excreted per 24 hours. Quantitative determination of excretion, to be useful, must be done on a _____ urine specimen.

339

hypo	Urine may be collected either as a *single-voided* specimen or as a *timed* collection. Two hours, 12 hours, and 24 hours are common periods used to collect the _____ urine specimen; however, any convenient moment may be used to collect the _____ urine specimen.
19	**20**
(rise)	Considering the bacterial growth curve in frame 77, you would expect the change in pH to occur after _____ .
83	**84**
pale blue (slate gray)	The normal poly has a purple nucleus, but the Sternheimer-Malbin positive poly has a _____ nucleus.
147	**148**

A. Squamous epithelial
B. Red blood
C. Red blood

(If you missed **B** *or* **C**, *review frames 167 to 173.)*

211

As water is removed from distal renal tubular urine, if the urine contains abundant protein, this protein may gel within the cylindrical tubules, forming casts. Circle three shapes the protein may take when this occurs. (These are longitudinal views.)

A.

B.

C.

D.

212

---

oval fat bodies

275

In Figure 6 on page 151, *low* power, unstained, the dark refractile cells are _____ bodies.

276

---

timed (24-hour)

339

Albumin in the urine is called _____ .
If there is marked loss of albumin in the urine, there will be a _____ in the plasma albumin concentration.

340

timed single-voided	If you want to know the rate of excretion of urine, you need to measure its total _____ and the _____ over which it is collected.
20	**21**
four hours	When urine is allowed to stand at room temperature more than _____ hours, the microscopic examination may lose validity because _____ may cause the urine to become _____ which may result in the _____ of formed elements.
84	**85**
pale blue	When stained with the Sternheimer-Malbin stain, the normal poly has purple cytoplasmic granules, while the Sternheimer-Malbin positive poly has _____ granules.
148	**149**

A, B, and D *(If you circled C, look up the shape of a renal tubule.)*	This precipitated protein, called hyaline, may be dislodged from the distal renal tubule or collecting duct and appear in the urine where it is called a _____ cast.
212	**213**
oval fat	Color Figure 30 on page 166 is an unstained low-power view. Identify the objects: *Under* **A.** _____ cell. *To right of* **B.** _____ . *At end of line* **C.** _____ . *At end of line* **D.** _____ . *At end of line* **E.** _____ .
276	**277**
albuminuria decrease (fall)	In the nephrotic syndrome, because of the albuminuria that is present, the specific gravity of the urine is _____ .
340	**341**

---

volume

time

The 24-hour urine collection is an example of a
_____ . This type
of collection is necessary to determine the
_____ of urine excretion.

21   22

---

four

bacterial growth

alkaline

destruction
(deterioration)

Check the following procedure you think best for
preservation of the urinary sediment in 30 ml urine
for microscopic examination:

A. Add eight drops of 10 percent formalin.
B. Heat to 80 C for 40 minutes.

85   86

---

slate gray

List the difference in nuclear staining between the
normal poly and the Sternheimer-Malbin positive
poly.

Normal:_____.
Sternheimer-Malbin positive: _____.

149   150

hyaline	Because the renal tubule serves as a mold, the protein gel formed within it is a _____ of the tubule.
213	**214**

A. Squamous epithelial B. Oval fat body C. Red blood cells D. Oval fat body E. Fat droplet	Notice that object **E**, color Figure 30, is a fat droplet. It may be differentiated from the cells at **C**, which are _____ cells, because its size is _____ and because it is more refractile.
277	**278**

increased (greater)	Actually, 0.4 g protein per 100 ml urine _____ the specific gravity 0.001. Therefore the specific gravity of the protein-free urine would be (higher) (lower).
341	**342**

timed collection rate	A patient being instructed in collecting a 24-hour urine specimen should be told to start at a convenient hour, such as 8:00 AM, empty his bladder and discard that urine, then save all urine up to and including that voided at _____ of the second day.
22	**23**
✓A. Add eight drops of 10 percent formalin	Both of these, that is, the addition of _____ and heating, kill bacteria, but the addition of_____ drops of _____ per 30 ml urine fixes the formed elements.
86	**87**

purple
 	
pale blue
	Now list the difference in staining of the cytoplasmic granules.
	   Normal: _____ .
	   Sternheimer-Malbin positive: _____ .

150	**151**

cast	Circle the shape that more nearly represents a cast. A. B. 214 215
red blood less (smaller)	The large object just below the center in color Figure 31, oil immersion, unstained, shows many _____ within a cell. Identify it.
278	279
raises (increases) lower	To calculate the specific gravity of protein-free urine, for every 0.4 g protein per 100 ml urine _____ must be _____ _____ the specific gravity reading.
342	343

8:00 AM (the same hour)	In order to determine the _____ of urine excretion, it is necessary to have a (timed) (single-voided) urine collection. (Circle the correct answer.)
23	**24**

formalin eight 10 percent formalin	Therefore, _____ added to _____ ml of urine is the best method of preservation for microscopic examination. Check two of the following methods that also preserve urine by inhibiting bacterial growth: A. Refrigerate at 4 C. B. Keep in a warm, dark place. C. Add 2 ml toluene.
87	**88**

purple slate gray	The Sternheimer-Malbin stain, because it stains other formed elements differentially, makes their identification (easier) (harder). (Circle the correct answer.)
151	**152**

A	A major characteristic of a cast is that its sides are nearly _____ .
215	**216**

fat droplets Oval fat body	Sometimes small fat droplets fuse into large fat droplets like **B** in Figure 2 on page 149, but the five objects out of focus in the upper left corner of color Figure 31 on page 167 are not as refractile as fat and are probably_____ .
279	**280**

0.001 subtracted from	A 24-hour urine having a volume of 2000 ml and containing 16 g protein gives a reading on the urinometer of 1.016. Its true specific gravity is _____ .
343	**344**

rate

timed

Put an "s" after those tests usually done on a single-voided urine specimen and a "t" after those that must be done on a timed collection:

Test for glucosuria _____.
24-hour protein excretion _____ .
Test for proteinuria _____.
Creatinine clearance _____ .

24   25

---

eight drops of
10 percent
formalin

30

√A. Refrigerate
        at 4 C
√C. Add 2 ml
        toluene

If urine is needed for chemical examination, bacterial growth is inhibited and the urine preserved, but the formed elements are not fixed, when ____ ml _____ are layered over the urine or when the urine is _____ at _____.

88   89

---

easier

The Sternheimer-Malbin stain is done on a (wet) (dry) preparation of a fresh urine sediment and is useful for the identification of _____ and other _____ .

152   153

parallel	In color Figure 12 on page 163, high power, stained, the large dark-purple object above the letter **B** is a _____ because its sides are nearly _____ .
216	**217**
red blood cells	In Figure 2 on page 149, **C** is a small, highly refractile_____ .
280	**281**
1.014	If one wishes to determine the specific gravity of urine from which the protein has been removed, the urine can be boiled; this causes the protein to _____ , and it can then be removed by filtration.
344	**345**

s

t

s

t

Two types of urine collections are used:

A. _____

B. _____

25 | 26

2

toluene

refrigerated

4 C

Bacterial growth is inhibited, the formed elements are fixed, and the urine is preserved when _____ are added per ____ ml urine.

89 | 90

(wet)

Sternheimer-
Malbin positive

polys

formed elements

The Sternheimer-Malbin positive _____ may show Brownian movement of its cytoplasmic granules (best seen with oil immersion lens) when the specific gravity of the urine is close to that of a protein-free plasma filtrate that has a specific gravity of _____ to _____.
Because of this they have been called "glitter cells."

153 | 154

cast parallel	Hyaline casts not containing inclusions are nearly transparent and therefore are seen best under reduced illumination. Circle the hyaline cast not containing inclusions. A. B. 217 218
fat droplet	Identify the following in color Figure 32 on page 167, high power, stained: A. _____ . *Below* B. _____ . *Below* C. _____ . *At end of line* D. _____ . 281 282
precipitate (be denatured or coagulate)	A common qualitative test for protein in the urine (sulfosalicylic acid) is based on the _____ of protein. 345 346

single-voided specimen

timed collection

Physical Examination of the Urine

Specific gravity is a measure of the weight of particles in solution. Specifically, it is the ratio of the weight of a given volume of fluid to the weight of the same volume of distilled water. Distilled water has a specific gravity of _____.

26

27

---

eight drops of 10 percent formalin

30

Preservation of urine may be done by

A. _____

B. _____

C. _____

(Check the method that is best for microscopic examination.)

90

91

---

poly

1.006

1.008

Besides the staining characteristics, Sternheimer-Malbin positive polys may show _____ _____ of the _____, if the specific gravity of the urine is about _____.

154

155

A

The large object in color Figure 13 on page 163 high power, unstained, although it has a few small inclusions, is predominantly a _____.

218

219

A. Oval fat body
B. Red blood cell
C. Large fat drop-
   let
D. Large fat drop-
   let

B differs from C and D in that C and D are more
_____ .

282

283

---

precipitation

In this test the degree of cloudiness (or amount of precipitate) is proportional to the _____ of protein present.

346

347

1.000	Specific gravity is a measure of the weight of particles in _____.
27	**28**

refrigeration at 4 C adding 2 ml toluene √adding eight drops 10 percent formalin per 30 ml urine	The probability of seeing formed elements in the urine increases with their _____ per unit volume of urine. Therefore, in very dilute urine the probability of seeing formed elements is (increased) (decreased). (Circle the correct answer.)
91	**92**

Brownian movement cytoplasmic granules 1.006 to 1.008	The Sternheimer-Malbin positive poly has the following characteristics: A. _____ nucleus. B. _____ cytoplasmic granules. C. _____ _____ _____
155	**156**

hyaline cast	Nearly all of the smaller elements in color Figure 13 are _____.
219	**220**
refractile	Color Figure 33 on page 167 is a stained high-power view. Cast **A** is predominantly a _____ cast, while cast **B** contains many refractile _____ and therefore is called a _____ cast.
283	**284**
concentration	A common qualitative test for proteinuria is _____. It is based upon _____.
347	**348**

solution

Specifically, specific gravity is the ratio of the weight of a given volume of fluid to the weight of the same volume of _____ .

28

29

---

number
(concentration)

decreased

When fluids are restricted for 12 hours, urine excreted by the normal person has a specific gravity above _____ . Therefore, in the first morning urine specimen you would expect to have a _____ chance of seeing formed elements.

92

93

A. Pale blue
B. Slate gray
C. Cytoplasmic granules showing Brownian movement if specific gravity is about 1.006 to 1.008.

"Glitter cells" are those Sternheimer-Malbin positive polys that show _____ of the cytoplasmic granules when the _____ _____ of the urine is about _____ _____ .

156

157

red blood cells	Casts are formed within the renal _____ and characteristically have_____ _____ .
220	**221**
hyaline fat droplets fatty	The fatty cast (**B**) in color Figure 33 contains refractile fat droplets that vary in their _____ .
284	**285**
sulfosalicylic acid the precipitation of protein	Bence Jones protein is an abnormal protein that is unusual in that at pH 5 it precipitates as urine is heated or cooled between 45 C and 70 C. But it will redissolve at boiling temperature and below 45 C. The usual protein in urine after boiling remains in a state of _____ .
348	**349**

distilled water

Specific gravity is a measure of the _____ of particles in solution.

29

30

1.022

better

In a urine that is dilute and therefore has a _____ specific gravity you would expect to see _____ formed elements than in a _____ urine.

93

94

Brownian move-
ment

specific gravity

1.006 to 1.008

Bacteria may be seen on an unstained urine sediment but are usually more clearly seen when it is _____.

157

158

tubule parallel sides	The presence of an occasional hyaline cast in the urinary sediment is normal; however, the finding of one or more hyaline casts per low-power field is _____ .
221	**222**
size	In Figure 14 on page 155, high power, unstained, the formed elements in the large group are _____, and the entire group is probably a _____ .
285	**286**
precipitation	Bence Jones protein has a relatively low molecular weight. It is found in the urine in many cases of multiple myeloma. Like albumin it is precipitated by _____ acid.
349	**350**

weight	Specific gravity is the ratio of the _____ of a given _____ to the _____ of the same _____ _____ .
30	**31**

low fewer concentrated	If red blood cells are present in urine that is more dilute than plasma, you would expect these red cells to _____ and finally _____ .
94	**95**

stained	To see bacteria to better advantage, the urine sediment can be dried on the slide, which may then be _____ .
158	**159**

abnormal	The number of hyaline casts that you can see in color Figure 14 on page 163, low power, unstained, is _____.
222	**223**
red blood cells red blood cell cast	Compared to the fat droplets in cast **B**, color Figure 33, the red cells in the cast in Figure 14 on page 155 are (more) (less) uniform in size and (more) (less) refractile.
286	**287**
sulfosalicylic	The presence of Bence Jones proteinuria should be confirmed by electrophoresis. As multiple myeloma is a cause of the nephrotic syndrome, the proteinuria of a patient with this disease may consist of both _____ and _____.
350	**351**

weight	Clinically, specific gravity is determined with a hydrometer that is called a *urinometer.* The specific gravity of urine is the ratio of _____
volume of fluid	
weight	_____
volume of dis- tilled water	to _____ _____ .
31	**32**

swell	Other cellular formed elements behave in a similar fashion to red cells; therefore, the probability of seeing intact formed elements in the urine following a large fluid load is_____ .
lyse	
95	**96**

stained	Drying makes red cells, white cells, and casts difficult to identify. However, by using Gram's stain, any _____ present in the dried sediment are more easily identified.
159	**160**

zero	Color Figure 15 on page 163 is a low-power view, unstained, of the same urine sediment. There is a predominantly_____ cast, which is visible because the illumination has been _____ .
223	**224**

(more) (less)	In Figure 15 on page 156, high power, unstained, this _____ is composed of _____ and is called a _____ .
287	**288**

Bence Jones protein albumin	In multiple myeloma a diagnostic finding is the presence of _____ in the urine, which is characterized by _____ .
351	**352**

the weight of a given volume of urine the weight of the same volume of distilled water	Clinically, a _____ is used to determine _____ . It is calibrated, usually at 20 C, to read 1.000 in _____ .
32	**33**
less	Two reasons for this decreased probability of seeing as many intact formed elements are A. they may be _____; B. they will be present in _____ numbers per unit volume.
96	**97**
bacteria	Stains of the dried urine sediment are most useful in identification of _____ .
160	**161**

hyaline reduced	The cell labeled **A** in color Figure 15 is a _____ .
224	225
cast fat droplets fatty cast	Identify objects **A** and **D** on color Figure 34 on page 167, unstained, oil immersion: A. _____ . D. _____ .
288	289
Bence Jones protein precipitation between 45 C and 70 C and redissolving at boiling temperature and below 45 C.	Albumin in the urine can be tested by _____ .
352	353

urinometer (hydrometer) specific gravity distilled water	The urinometer is calibrated usually at _____C to read _____ .
33	**34**
A. disrupted B. decreased	The probability of seeing formed elements increases with their _____ per unit volume of urine. This probability is greater with the first morning urine specimen, which has a higher specific gravity and a _____ volume.
97	**98**
bacteria	To identify the *tubercle bacillus* in the urinary sediment, an _____ stain is done on the _____ urine sediment.
161	**162**

red blood cell	Look at color Figure 16 on page 164, a low-power view of a urine sediment stained with the Stern-heimer-Malbin stain. This stain makes the formed elements more visible, especially ones like C, which is a _____ .
225	226

A. Red blood cell D. Red blood cell	In color Figure 34 the object at the end of the line from B is a fat droplet. The cast, C, is composed of _____ . Therefore this is a _____ cast.
289	290

sulfosalicylic acid	Hemoglobin is another protein that may be present in the urine in abnormal states. Whereas hematuria may be detected by microscopic examination, hemoglobinuria must be determined by a _____ .
353	354

20 1.000 in dis- tilled water	One reads from the stem of the freely floating urinometer at the lowest point of the curving meniscus of the surface of the urine. Draw a line where one takes the reading. 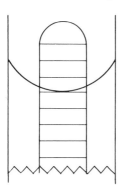
34	**35**
number (concentration) smaller	In microscopic examination of the urine, you are concerned with enumeration of the formed elements in the urinary sediment. Since, usually, few formed elements are excreted in the urine each day, it is useful to _____ them by centrifugation before the urinary sediment is examined.
98	**99**
acid-fast (Ziehl-Neelsen) dried	*E. coli* and staphylococci are best stained with _____ stain.
162	**163**

hyaline cast

|

Identify the other labeled formed elements in color Figure 16 (low power). Note that cell **A** has folded cytoplasm.

A. _____ cell.

B. _____ .

226

227

---

fat droplets

fatty

|

In Figure 1 on page 149, low power, unstained, there is an object with sides that are relatively _____. This (is) (is not) a cast.

290

291

---

chemical test

|

The benzidine test is commonly used to detect the presence of hemoglobin. Of course _____ _____ cells will give a positive test.

354

355

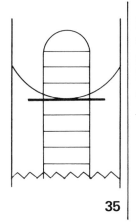

In the temperature range under consideration, water expands as the temperature rises. To the reading of the urinometer one *adds* 0.001 for each 3 C that the urine is *above* the calibration temperature and _____ for each _____ C that it is below.

35

36

concentrate

Since the urinary sediment is _____ than the urine in which it is suspended, it will settle to the _____ of the urine specimen bottle.

99

100

Gram's

The presence of bacteria in a dried preparation of urine sediment is easily determined by the use of methylene _____ stain.

163

164

A. Squamous epithelial

(If you missed this, go back to frame 187.)

B. Hyaline cast

227

A plain hyaline cast contains no inclusions within the matrix. Circle the plain hyaline casts.

A.

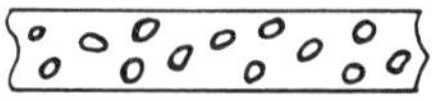

B.

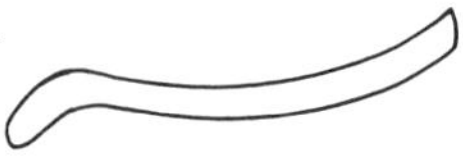

C.

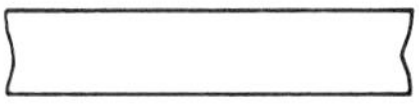

D.

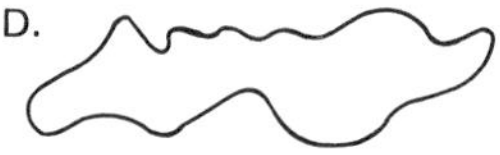

228

---

parallel

~~is not~~

291

If you said that this is not a cast, you were correct, because casts (are) (are not) made of fibrous strands.

292

---

red blood

355

Hematuria is verified _____ . Hemoglobinuria is determined by the _____ test.

356

subtracts 0.001

3

A freshly voided urine, now at 32 C, gives a reading of 1.018 on a urinometer. What is its true specific gravity (at 20 C)?

36

37

---

heavier (denser)

bottom

Because of this, before a 12 ml aliquot of urine is removed from the urine in the specimen bottle for centrifugation at 1500 rpm for five minutes, the urine should be thoroughly _____ .

100

101

---

blue

Wright's stain is commonly used for studying red and white cells on dried blood films. Neutrophils and eosinophils in dried urinary sediment can be identified by the use of _____ stain.

164

165

B and C	If you circled D, you were in error because the sides are not _____ .
228	**229**

(are not)	This object (is) (is not) a contaminant and is a _____ .
292	**293**

microscopically benzidine	The most common sugar found in the urine is glucose (glucosuria). However, rarely, fructose or other sugars may be present. In diabetes mellitus a urine specific gravity greater than 1.030 may be seen when there is _____ .
356	**357**

1.022

A urine taken from the refrigerator, now at 11 C, gives a reading of 1.015 on a urinometer. What is its true specific gravity?

37

38

mixed

The urine sediment is concentrated for microscopic examination by _____ of a _____ ml aliquot of urine at _____ rpm for _____ minutes.

101

102

Wright's

Four stains done on dried urine sediments are:

A. _____ stain.
B. _____ stain.
C. _____ stain.
D. _____ stain.

165

166

parallel

While cellular hyaline casts have a hyaline matrix, they are called cellular casts because they also contain _____ . Label these casts.

A._____ cast.   B. _____ cast.

229

230

(is)

fiber

With *trichomonas vaginalis* infestation the urine may be contaminated with the motile parasite _____ .

293

294

---

glucosuria

0.27 g glucose per 100 ml urine elevates the specific gravity of the urine 0.001. In diabetes mellitus when glucosuria is present the specific gravity of the urine will be (increased) (decreased).

357

358

1.012

38

The kidney conserves water by concentrating urine or loses water from the body by diluting the urine. The kidney of a normal subject, under conditions of restricted fluid intake for 12 hours, can _____ urine to a specific gravity greater than 1.022 and, with sufficiently increased water intake, can _____ urine to a specific gravity less than 1.005. In renal disease there is inability to _____ or _____ the urine to the normal extent.

39

---

centrifugation

12

1500

five

102

After centrifugation of a _____ ml aliquot of urine at _____ for _____ minutes, 11.5 ml of the supernatant solution is poured off, and uniform resuspension of the _____ is again accomplished in the remaining _____ ml urine.

103

Gram's

Acid-fast

Methylene blue

Wright's

166

Other than bacteria and yeasts, the smallest cells found in the urinary sediment are seen in color Figure 3, on page 161, high power, unstained. Identify them.

167

cells A. Cellular B. Hyaline	Look at color Figure 17 on page 164, high power, stained. The large cast in the right upper quadrant is obviously a _____ cast.
230	**231**
trichomonas *vaginalis*	*Trichomonas* parasites have a flagellum and are easily recognized when alive because they are _____ .
294	**295**
(increased)	Therefore, for every 0.27 g glucose per 100 ml urine, 0.001 should be (added to) (subtracted from) the specific gravity reading to calculate the specific gravity of the urine if free of glucose.
358	**359**

concentrate dilute concentrate dilute **39**	After 12 hours of fluid restriction, the normal kidney can concentrate urine to a specific gravity above _____, and after ample water ingestion, it can dilute urine to a specific gravity under _____ . **40**
12 1500 rpm five sediment 0.5 **103**	Since the urinary sediment is so compacted at the bottom of the tube by centrifugation, uniform resuspension of the _____ must be accomplished by (gently) (vigorously) flicking the bottom of the centrifuge tube ten times. (Circle the correct answer.) **104**
Red blood cells **167**	Do all the cells in this slide look exactly the same size? **168**

cellular	Sometimes it is difficult to classify casts. The formed element in color Figure 18 on page 164, low-power, stained, is primarily a _____ cast.
231	**232**
motile	When *trichomonas* parasites die they may resemble a renal tubular epithelial cell. A distinguishing feature of the *trichomonas* is the presence of a _____ .
295	**296**
(subtracted from)	A 24-hour urine has a volume of 2000 ml and contains 21.6 g glucose. The urinometer reads 1.014. The actual specific gravity of the urine if free of sugar would be _____ .
359	**360**

1.022 1.005	One of the early changes in kidney function seen in arteriolar nephrosclerosis of hypertensive vascular disease is the loss of ability to _____ or _____ the urine.
40	**41**
sediment (vigorously)	Since one drop of this resuspended urine sediment will be examined under the microscope, to be truly representative of the entire specimen, it must be _____ resuspended.
104	**105**
No	Some red blood cells appear as if they were in a hypotonic solution (that is, they are _____), while others appear crenated (with irregular spiny surfaces), as if they were in a _____ solution.
168	**169**

hyaline

(A cast should contain several cells before you call it a cellular cast.)

232

Here are two groups of cells as you might find them in urine. One is a cluster, and the other is a _____ cast. Circle the latter.

A.

B.

233

---

flagellum

296

Sperm can be recognized by their short heads and long _____ .

297

1.010

360

One common test for glucosuria utilizes glucose oxidase impregnated paper. This is specific for

_____ .

361

concentrate dilute	In renal disease the specific gravity of the urine may become "fixed" at or near 1.010, which is slightly higher than the specific gravity of a protein-free filtrate of plasma. A "fixed" specific gravity is evidence that the kidney has lost the ability to _____ _____ .
41	**42**
uniformly	It is for this reason that the centrifuge tube is _____ flicked _____ times.
105	**106**
swollen (larger) hypertonic	After ample water ingestion the normal individual can dilute urine to a specific gravity under _____ . Red cells in such urine will _____ and may _____ .
169	**170**

cellular
A

It is a cellular cast because it has

A. _____.
B. _____.

233 | 234

---

tails

In Figure 16 on page 156, high power, stained, there are three _____ present.

297 | 298

---

glucose

Ketones (acetoacetic acid, acetone, and β-hydroxybutyric acid) appear in the urine (ketonuria) when carbohydrate metabolism is deficient, such as in starvation or poorly controlled diabetes mellitus. In following patients being treated for diabetic acidosis, it is useful to test urine for both _____ and _____.

361 | 362

concentrate or dilute the urine	In renal disease, with loss of ability of the kidney to concentrate or dilute, the specific gravity of the urine approaches _____ .
42	43
vigorously ten	One common error in preparation of the urine sediment after centrifugation is the failure to resuspend the sediment _____ by flicking the centrifuge tube _____ times.
106	107
1.005 swell lyse	Red blood cells with irregular spiny surfaces are _____ red cells.
170	171

parallel sides cellular inclu- sions	Color Figure 19, page 164, is a high-power view of an unstained urine sediment. Identify: A. _____ cell. B. _____ cell.
234	**235**
sperm	Figure 17 on page 157 is an unstained high power view. Cell **A**, which is partially obscured by debris, is a red blood cell. Identify **B**.
298	**299**
glucose ketones	The ketones found in urine when carbohydrate metabolism is deranged are A. _____ . B. _____ . C. _____ .
362	**363**

1.010	The osmolality of a protein-free filtrate of plasma is approximately 310 mOsm/kg water. In contrast to specific gravity, osmolality is a determination of more physiologic significance because it measures the *number* of particles in solution, while specific gravity is a measure of the _____ _____ .
43	**44**

uniformly vigorously ten	Certain formed elements in the urinary sediment, such as hyaline casts, are difficult to visualize under an ordinary amount of light because they transmit light almost as well as the surrounding urine. Therefore, to see hyaline casts and similar formed elements, the light must be (increased) (reduced). (Circle the correct answer.)
107	**108**

crenated	The number of crenated red blood cells clearly seen in color Figure 3 is (zero) (one) (six) (twelve). (Circle the correct answer.)
171	**172**

A. Red blood B. Red blood	The large group of compacted small cells just below the center of color Figure 19 is most likely a cast composed of _____ cells.
235	236
Trichomonas	The object **B** (is) (is not) a renal tubular epithelial cell because it has a _____ , and it (does) (does not) have a prominent nucleus.
299	300
acetoacetic acid acetone β-hydroxybutyric acid	Another ketone found in the urine when there is a specific metabolic defect is phenylpyruvic acid (phenylketonuria). It can be detected with Phenistix®. As this metabolic defect, if untreated, results in brain damage, it is important to check all infants' urines for _____ .
363	364

weight of particles in solution	The osmotic movement of water across the renal tubule is governed by the _____ of particles in solution rather than by their _____ .
44	**45**

(reduced)	In Figure 3 on page 150 (a high-power view) there are formed elements present. Can you identify them? (yes) (no)
108	**109**

(one)	In color Figure 4, on page 161, high power, unstained, the group of small nonnucleated cells, similar to cell B and cell C, are _____ cells.
172	**173**

red blood

(If you thought these were polys, look at the polys in Figure 9 on page 137, high power, unstained.)

236

In contrast to cells **A** and **B** (color Figure 19), cells **C** and **D** are _____ in size. They could be more easily identified by using a _____ .

237

---

is not

flagellum

does not

300

In color Figure 35 on page 167, high power, Sternheimer-Malbin stain, identify the following:

A. _____ .
B. _____ .
C. _____ .

301

---

phenylpyruvic acid

364

Phenylketonuria is determined by means of _____ .

365

number

weight

45

Osmolality is a measure of _____ _____ per kg of water.

46

(no)

109

The same formed elements are in Figure 4 on page 150 (a high-power view). Can you identify them? (yes) (no)

110

---

red blood

173

In addition to sometimes seeing bacteria and red blood cells in the urine of a patient with an acute urinary tract infection, what other cell would you expect to see?

174

larger

stain

237	

On the basis of their size, cells **C** and **D** in color Figure 19 could be either _____ _____ cells or _____ .

238

A. Red blood cell
B. Poly (normal)
C. Bacteria

301

With the Sternheimer-Malbin stain, live bacteria do not stain, but dead _____ stain a _____ color.

302

Phenistix®

365

Bilirubin in the urine (bilirubinuria) causes the *foam* of urine that has been shaken to be colored yellow or brown. The foam test is the simplest way to check for _____ .

366

the number of
particles

46

Which measurement of renal concentrating and diluting ability has more physiologic significance?

A. Specific gravity
B. Osmolality

(Check the correct answer.)

                                                        47

(yes)

110

These formed elements are cells. They are easily identified as _____cells because they lack nuclei.

111

---

poly
(polymorpho-
nuclear
leukocyte)

174

The poly is usually (larger) (smaller) than the red blood cell and contains a _____ .

175

renal tubular epithelial	Color Figure 20 on page 164 is a stained, high-power view. Identify:
polys	A. _____ cell.
	B. _____ cell.
238	**239**

bacteria	Go back to Figure 9 on page 153, unstained, low power. If you look closely you will see that
purple	between the clumps of _____ there are _____ present.
302	**303**

bilirubinuria	Urine is screened for bilirubin by the _____ test. Its presence is then confirmed by more specific tests.
366	**367**

√B. Osmolality

An ionized substance, such as sodium chloride, because it contributes two particles (ions) to a solution, has a much greater effect on _____ than it has on _____
_____.

47

48

red blood

Too much light made the formed elements invisible in Figure 3; however, they became visible in Figure 4 when the light was _____.

111

112

larger

nucleus

There are (one) (six) (ten) red blood cells that are clearly identifiable in color Figure 1, on page 161.

175

176

A. Red blood B. Renal tubular epithelial *(If you missed* B, *look at frames* *192 and 193.)*	On color Figure 20 also identify: C. _____ . D. _____ .
239	**240**
polys bacteria	Bacteria may be seen in a stained or _____ urine sediment, but more precise identification is obtained if the urine sediment is _____ on a slide and stained with _____ stain.
303	**304**
foam	The Phenistix® test is used to detect _____ .
367	**368**

osmolality

specific gravity

A 150 millimol per kg water solution of urea has an osmolality that is (greater than) (about the same as) (less than) a 150 mM/kg water solution of sodium chloride.

(Circle the correct answer.)

48

49

reduced

Therefore, one *error* to be avoided in examining urine sediments is the use of _____ _____.

112

113

(six)

How many polys are there in this slide?

176

177

C. Cellular cast (renal tubular epithelial cell cast) D. Red blood cell	In the right-upper quadrant of color Figure 17 on page 164, stained, high power, there is a _____ cast. Cells marked **A** are _____ cells. The cell marked **B** is a _____ .
240	**241**

unstained dried Gram's	Of course, the *tubercle bacillus* is stained with _____ .
304	**305**

phenylketonuria	**Bacteriologic Examination of the Urine** Detection of urinary tract infection is extremely important and can be done on a *clean voided* urine specimen. Catheterization is not necessary. White blood cells (polys) and bacteria are usually found in the centrifuged sediment of the urine when urinary tract _____ is present.
368	**369**

(less than)

The normal kidney after 12 hours of fluid restriction can concentrate urine to a specific gravity greater than _____ (or to an osmolality greater than 850 mOsm/kg water) and can dilute urine after sufficient water ingestion to a specific gravity of_____ or less (an osmolality usually less than 250 mOsm/kg water).

49   **50**

---

too much light

Since some formed elements, such as casts, are much larger than white or red blood cells, they are more easily counted using (high-) (low-) power magnification.

(Circle the correct answer.)

113   **114**

One

Notice that this poly is stained with the Stern-heimer-Malbin stain, which stains the nucleus _____ and the cytoplasmic granules _____ .

177   **178**

cellular red blood poly	Although the other cells in this cast are not as easily identified as cell **B**, they are probably the same, and this cast is therefore composed of _____ .
241	**242**
acid-fast stain (Ziehl-Neelsen)	Salts that commonly precipitate out in the urine are _____ and _____ .
305	**306**
infection	For determining the presence or absence of bacteria in the dried urinary sediment, a simpler stain than the Gram stain, that is, the _____ stain, may be used.
369	**370**

1.022

1.005

Urine, which is isosmolal to a protein-free filtrate of plasma (about _____ mOsm/kg water), usually has a specific gravity of 1.006 to 1.008. Therefore, a "fixed" urinary specific gravity of 1.010 actually represents (no) (some) (considerable) renal concentrating ability.

(Circle the correct answer.)

50

51

(low-)

Casts are reported as the average number per _____ power field.

114

115

---

purple

purple

This staining is characteristic of the _____ poly.

178

179

polys	This cellular cast, composed of polys (white blood cells), is commonly called a _____ blood cell cast.
242	**243**
phosphates urates	Urates are usually present in an amorphous form. Since uric acid is relatively insoluble in acid urine, crystals of _____ are only seen when the urine is _____.
306	**307**
methylene blue	To further characterize the nature of any bacteria present, a _____ stain should be done on the _____ urinary sediment.
370	**371**

310

(some)

51

Although specific gravity is more commonly determined, osmolality is a measurement having more _____ significance.

52

low-

115

To count cellular elements, _____ power magnification is used, and they are reported as the average number per _____

_____.

116

normal

179

The renal tubular epithelial cell is about the size of a poly but has different morphology.

Cell A is a _____.
Cell B is a _____.

A.   B.

180

white	In color Figure 21 on page 165, stained, oil immersion, the predominant cell nucleus is not multilobulated; therefore, this is a _____ _____.
243	**244**
uric acid acidic	Uric acid crystals are plate-like and irregular in shape in contrast to calcium oxalate crystals, which are _____ in shape.
307	**308**
Gram dried	Polys are looked for in the sediment of the _____ freshly voided urine specimen. If polys are found in clumps, it is very suggestive that _____ is present.
371	**372**

physiologic	The gross appearance of urine may provide important clues to the presence of abnormality. However, urine that appears turbid or cloudy on _____ examination may be normal on microscopic examination.
52	**53**

high high-power field	Compared to the low-power magnification, with the high-power magnification _____ the number of white and red blood cells seen in any one field.
116	**117**

A. poly B. renal tubular epithelial cell	Identify the grouped cells in color Figure 5 on page 161, high power, stained.
180	**181**

renal tubular epithelial cell cast	Cellular casts indicate the presence of a renal abnormality. Three types of cells which may be in casts are A. _____. B. _____. C. _____.
244	245

regular	Label the following crystals: A. B.
308	309

clean urinary tract infection	Bacteria are characterized by examining a _____ stain of the (wet) (dried) urine sediment of a _____ freshly voided urine specimen.
372	373

gross

Conversely, urine that appears clear on gross examination may show many _____ findings on _____ examination.

53 | 54

reduces

Therefore, the urine sediment should first be examined under _____ magnification to enumerate casts and then examined under _____ magnification to enumerate _____ _____ .

117 | 118

Renal tubular epithelial cells

Identify cells **A** and **B** stained with the Sternheimer-Malbin stain in color Figure 2 on page 161, high power

A. _____ .
B. _____ .

181 | 182

red blood cells polys (WBCs) renal tubular epithelial cells	Red cell casts and white cell casts should be specified as such. The term "cellular cast" is commonly used to designate a _____ _____ cast.
245	246

A. Uric acid B. Calcium oxalate	Phosphate precipitates in alkaline urine; therefore, crystals of triple _____ may be seen when the urine is _____. (Triple refers to the magnesium ammonium salt.)
309	310

Gram (dried) clean	If bacteria are readily found on Gram stain of the sediment, it is likely that _____ _____ is present.
373	374

abnormal

microscopic

54

If urine contains sufficient suspended precipitated salts, white cells, or red cells, it may appear _____ on gross examination.

55

---

low-power

high-power

white and red blood cells (smaller formed elements)

118

In distinguishing the abnormal urinary sediment from the normal, it is necessary to enumerate the casts per _____ power field and cells per _____ power field.

119

A. Renal tubular epithelial cell
B. Poly

182

In this figure, cell **B** is a (Sternheimer-Malbin positive) (normal) poly because it meets the following criteria:

A. _____ .
B. _____ .

183

renal tubular epithelial cell	Hyaline casts which taper at one end are sometimes called cylindroids. Label these casts. A. ⊐_____⊏ _____ B. ⊐_____⊐ _____ **247**
246	

phosphate alkaline	Name this crystal found in an alkaline urine. **311**
310	

urinary tract infection	It is not necessary to catheterize patients unless they are unable to cooperate in providing _____ urine specimens. **375**
374	

turbid (cloudy or colored)	Microscopic examination is the only way to find out the reason for turbidity or cloudiness noted on _____ examination.
55	**56**
low- high-	An error to be avoided when examining the urine sediment is the failure to use both _____ _____ power magnifications.
119	**120**
Sternheimer- Malbin positive Pale blue nucleus Slate gray cyto- plasmic granules	Although their nuclei are nearly the same size, lower urinary tract transitional epithelial cells have more cytoplasm than renal tubular epithelial cells and are therefore _____ than renal tubular epithelial cells.
183	**184**

A. Hyaline cast
B. Cylindroid

Figure 11 on page 154, stained, is a low-power view of a cast that, although containing some inclusions, is primarily a _____ cast. Because it tapers at one end it may be called a

_____ .

247 | 248

Triple phosphate

The crystals shown in Figure 18 on page 157, low power, stained, are not shaped like but are shaped like _____ . (Draw shape.) They are therefore crystals of _____ .

311 | 312

---

clean voided

If active infection in the urinary tract is clinically apparent, usually there will be more than 100,000 colonies of bacteria present per ml urine on the culture of a _____ urine specimen.

375 | 376

gross

On gross examination urine may appear turbid or cloudy because of the presence of

A. _____ salts,
B. _____ cells, or
C. _____ cells.

56   57

---

high- and low-

Look at Figure 5 and Figure 6, both on page 151 (both low-power views). One of these is of a urine collected in a bedpan contaminated by mineral oil, and the other is of a urine from a nephrotic patient who has fat droplets in the urine. The dark refractile material is lipid. Can you distinguish which one is from the nephrotic patient and which one contains the foreign material? (yes) (no)

120   121

---

larger

Look carefully at the number of nuclear lobes in each cell. Identify the following in color Figure 6 on page 162, stained, low power:

Cell **A.** _____ .
Cell below **B.** _____ .
Cell **C.** _____ .

184   185

hyaline cylindroid	In renal failure, casts may form in large, dilated tubules. In contrast to narrow casts, renal failure casts are _____ .
248	**249**

  calcium oxalate	The crystals seen in Figure 19 on page 158, low power, stained, are _____ crystals.
312	**313**

clean voided	When urinary tract infection is less active, or after suppressive treatment has been given, there may be _____ 100,000 colonies of bacteria per ml urine.
376	**377**

A. precipitated
B. white
C. red

The reason for urine being turbid or cloudy or having a sediment can only be determined by _____ examination.

57

58

---

no

In collecting urine, an error to avoid is the _____ of the specimen by oils, fibers, or other _____ materials.

121

122

A. Renal tubular epithelial cell
B. Transitional epithelial cell
C. Poly (note that its nucleus has three lobes)

In color Figure 6 the pale cell below and to the right of the letter C is a _____ .

185

186

broad	Figure 12 on page 154 is an unstained low-power view. B is a waxy cast. Identify A.
249	**250**

uric acid	The crystals in Figure 20 on page 158, high power, stained, appeared in an alkaline urine. Name them.
313	**314**

less than	It is then necessary to get two or three urine cultures to see whether the same organism is consistently present in the urine. If it is, this organism is likely to be significant as the agent causing the _____.
377	**378**

microscopic	Phosphates and urates are salts that commonly precipitate out in urine and make it appear _____.
58	**59**
contamination foreign	If the urine specimen remains too long on the slide so that it is allowed to dry, the formed elements are (easier) (harder) to identify.
122	**123**
red blood cell	The squamous epithelial cell has more cytoplasm than the transitional epithelial cell and has a more irregular outline, as shown by cell **D**. Identify the following cells in color Figure 7 on page 162, high power, stained: A. _____. B. _____. C. _____.
186	**187**

Squamous epithelial cell	Cast **B**, Figure 12, is approximately as wide as the diameter of a squamous epithelial cell. It is a (broad) (narrow) cast.
250	**251**
Triple phosphate	In cystinuria, hexagonal crystals of _____ may appear in the urine.
314	**315**
urinary tract infection	When infection in the kidney (pyelonephritis) is active, there is usually some proteinuria in addition to having _____ and _____ in the urine sediment. The nuclei of these _____ will stain _____ with the Sternheimer-Malbin stain.
378	**379**

turbid (cloudy)

The turbidity or cloudiness due to a
_____ of urate or phosphate salts
can usually be distinguished from the turbidity
due to the presence of red blood cells, because
a moderate number of red cells makes the urine
smoky or opalescent.

59

60

(harder)

Therefore, one error in examining the urine
sediment is allowing it to _____ on
the slide.

123

124

A. Red blood
   cell
B. Squamous
   epithelial cell
C. Poly

Look at color Figure 7. In addition to cell B, how
many other squamous epithelial cells are there?
(one) (four) six)

187

188

(broad)	Identify the following in color Figure 22 on page 165, low power, stained. A. _____cast. B. _____ cell. C. _____ cell.
251	**252**
cystine	The crystals seen in Figure 21 on page 159, unstained, low power, are _____ crystals which are easily identified because of their _____ shape.
315	**316**
polys bacteria polys pale blue	Such a patient with pyelonephritis may have loss of renal tubular concentrating ability; therefore, fluid restriction for 12 hours may not result in a urine specific gravity greater than _____ .
379	**380**

precipitate	The precipitated salts commonly found in urine are _____ or _____ .
60	**61**
dry	One error in collecting the urine is allowing it to be _____ by _____ material.
124	**125**
(four)	In this figure, cell **C** is a (Sternheimer-Malbin positive) (normal) poly.
188	**189**

A. Broad hyaline B. Squamous epithelial C. Red blood	In time the cells in a cellular cast degenerate into coarse granules, and the cast is then called a _____ granular cast.
252	253

cystine hexagonal	Label the calcium oxalate crystal "A," the uric acid crystal "B," the triple phosphate crystal "C," and the cystine crystal "D."
316	317

1.022	Pyuria and bacteriuria without proteinuria suggest (upper) (lower) urinary tract infection.
380	381

phosphates urates	A moderate number of red cells in urine may make it appear _____ or _____ .
61	**62**

contaminated foreign	One error in preparation of the urine sediment for microscopic examination is failure to _____ the sediment adequately.
125	**126**

Sternheimer- Malbin positive	In active urinary tract infections, one usually finds an increased number of _____ in the urinary sediment. The majority of these are _____ polys.
189	**190**

coarse

Fine granules in casts result from further degeneration, and then the casts appear in the urine as _____ casts.

253

254

B, C, A, D

Identify the following on color Figure 36 on page 168, stained, oil immersion:

A. _____ .

B. _____ .

317

318

---

lower

When the bacterial agent causing chronic urinary tract infection is elusive, or when unexplained microscopic hematuria is present, think of tuberculosis as the cause. Culture for tubercle bacilli should be done on sediment from a large volume of urine, such as a _____ urine collection.

381

382

smoky (turbid) opalescent (cloudy) **62**	If there are *many* red cells in the urine (hematuria), or if there is much hemoglobin (hemoglobinuria), urine will be reddish or brownish. A red or brown color of the urine is therefore a "tip" that it may contain _____ or _____ . **63**
resuspend **126**	Two errors in the microscopic examination of the urinary sediment are the use of _____ light and failure to use both _____ _____ . **127**
polys Sternheimer- Malbin positive **190**	In active urinary tract infections, one will also usually find _____ on a stained smear of the dried urine sediment. **191**

fine granular	Color Figure 23 on page 165 is an unstained high-power view. Cells labeled **A** are probably renal tubular epithelial cells. **B** is a _____.
254	**255**

A. Normal poly **B.** Bacteria	Identify on color Figure 37 on page 168, stained, high power: A. _____. B. _____. C. _____. D. _____.
318	**319**

24-hour	In addition to culturing for *tubercle bacilli*, one should do the _____ stain on the _____ urinary sediment.
382	**383**

red cells	Blood in the urine is called _____.
hemoglobin	*Return to page 1, answer frame 64.*
63	**64**

too much	Common errors in collection, preparation, and examination of the urine sediment are
high- and low-power magnifications	A. _____.
	B. _____.
	C. _____.
	D. _____.
	E. _____.
	Return to page 1, answer frame 128.
127	**128**

bacteria	Color Figure 8 on page 162 is a stained, low-power view of a group of_____.
	Return to page 2, answer frame 192.
191	**192**

coarse granular
cast

Figure 13 on page 155 is another unstained high-power view. Identify

A. _____ cell.

B. _____ cast.

Return to page 2, answer frame 256.

255

256

A. Squamous
    epithelial cell
B. Red blood cell
C. Sternheimer-
    Malbin positive
    poly
D. Red blood cell

Identify the following on color Figure 38 on page 168, high power, unstained:

Just below A. _____ .

End of line B. _____ .

Above the letter C is a group of cells constituting a

_____ :

D. _____ .

Return to page 2, answer frame 320.

319

320

---

acid-fast
(Ziehl-Neelsen)

dried

Congratulations! Now you know how to examine the urine.

In Part 2 you will find the methods for the tests used in examining the urine.

383

384

PART 2

methods for
examination
of the urine

methods for examination of the urine

A. Collection and Preservation of the Urine

1. Collection of a 24-hour Urine Specimen

a. Have the patient completely empty the urinary bladder and discard this urine exactly at the beginning of the 24-hour timed collection (such as 7:00 AM).

b. Collect all urine voided during the subsequent 24 hours, including that voided exactly at the end of the 24-hour period (such as 7:00 AM of the second day).

c. All urine collected must be refrigerated or preserved if analyses for perishable substances in it are to be performed.

2. Methods for Preservation of the Urine

a. Refrigeration of the urine at 4 C.

b. Addition of 2 ml toluene to the urine specimen.

c. Addition of eight drops of 10 percent formalin per 30 ml urine.

B. Methods for Examination of the Urinary Sediment

1. Examination of the Unstained Urine Sediment

Centrifuge 12 ml of fresh urine at 1500 rpm for five minutes in a conical test tube. Decant 11.5 ml from the tube and resuspend the sediment thoroughly in the remaining 0.5 ml of urine by vigorously flicking the bottom of the test tube ten times. Transfer a drop of the resuspended sediment to a clean microscope slide and cover it with a coverslip. Examine it microscopically under *reduced* illumination, first using low power, then high power. Enumerate the formed elements seen as the number per low- or high-power field.

2. The Sternheimer-Malbin Stain for Urine Sediment

a. Composition of the Stain.
Solution I:

Crystal violet	3.0 g
95 percent ethyl alcohol	20.0 cc
Ammonium oxalate	0.8 g
Triple distilled water	80.0 cc

Solution II:

Safranin 0	0.25 g
95 percent alcohol	10.0 cc
Triple distilled water	100.0 cc

b. Method for Using the Stain.
Three parts of Solution I are mixed with 97 parts of Solution II and the resultant mixture is then filtered. This solution stains satisfactorily within a pH range of 4 to 8. In highly alkaline solutions, the stain will precipitate. Make up a mixture of fresh stain every three months. In the interim, if precipitation of the stain occurs, filter it again. Centrifuge 12 ml of urine at 1500 rpm for five minutes in a conical tube. Decant 11.5 ml urine from the tube and resuspend the sediment thoroughly in the remaining 0.5 ml urine. Add two drops of stain to the 0.5 ml of resuspended urine sediment in the tube. Place a drop of the stained sediment on a microscope slide and cover it with a thin coverslip. This preparation may be examined with low and high power, as well as with the oil immersion lens of the microscope.

c. Observations
Red blood cells take up very little stain and are usually a faint pink color, but occasionally they stain more deeply. Yeast cells stain purple. This difference in staining is useful in differentiating red cells and yeasts. White cells and epithelial cells stain readily. The nuclei of

epithelial cells stain red or purple. The nuclei of polymorphonuclear leukocytes stain either deep red to purple or a pale blue. The polys containing dark red or purple nuclei have purple granules in their cytoplasm, and they are usually of uniform size. They occur commonly in lower urinary tract infection without renal involvement. The polymorphonuclear leukocytes having blue-staining nuclei are either small and have a glassy appearance with an indistinct nucleus, or, more frequently, they appear swollen, are much larger than ordinary leukocytes and have a tendency to variability in size and shape, to vacuolation and to extrusion of fragments of cytoplasm. The blue-staining nucleus in such a swollen cell is less discrete and is either multilobulated or divided into one to four spherical nuclei. The cytoplasmic granules of these cells stain slate gray and, when studied with the oil immersion lens, may show marked Brownian movement if the urine is isotonic. These swollen, pale blue-staining cells with slate gray granules are round, oval, or pear shaped. They are present in inflammatory renal diseases, particularly in pyelonephritis. When they do show Brownian movement of the cytoplasmic granules, they are sometimes called "glitter cells." Hyaline casts stain a pale pink to red. Granular elements in casts stain reddish, violet, or bluish in contrast to the relatively unstained, bright and shiny-appearing fat droplets of fatty casts. Fatty cells present a brilliantly refractile honeycomb-like structure in a slightly stained matrix. Bacteria stain a dark purple when dead and are either unstained or pink when living and active. Mycelia and spores of fungi appear light and purple. *Trichomonas hominis* parasites are either colorless or pale blue.

d. Reference.
Sternheimer R, Malbin B: Clinical recognition of pyelonephritis, with a new stain for urinary sediments. Am J Med 11:312, 1951

C. Substances Imparting Color to the Urine

Color	Substance
Yellow to amber	Bilirubin Nitrofurantin and derivatives Quinacrine (Atabrine®) Salicylazosulfapyridine (Azulfidine®)–in alkaline urine. Urobilin
Orange to red	Pyridium®
Brown to red	Hemoglobin Red blood cells
Red	Diphenylhydantoin (Dilantin®) Porphyrins Phenosulfonphthalein, bromsulfalein, or phenolphthalein in alkaline urine Pigment from beets
Blue to green	Amitriptyline (Elavil®) Methylene blue Biliverdin Acriflavine
Brown to black	Homogentisic acid Melanin Phenol Porphobilin Methyldopa (Aldomet®) Metronidazole (Flagyl®) Quinine
Pale blue fluorescence	Triamterene (Dyrenium®)

D. Methods for Chemical Examination of the Urine

1. Specific Gravity

a. Fill the urinometer tube nearly full of urine, but leaving sufficient room for the urinometer float.

b. Use only a urinometer that has been checked for accuracy against distilled water to read 1.000 at its calibration temperature. Make sure that the float does not touch the sides of the tube by gently twirling its stem.

c. Read the scale of the urinometer where it is intersected by the lowest portion of the curve of the meniscus of the surface of the urine. Interpolate to the nearest 0.001 unit.

d. If the urine is warm, ie, recently at body temperature, or is cold, ie, recently taken from the refrigerator, the specific gravity reading must be corrected. Use a thermometer to determine the actual urine temperature. Add 0.001 to the specific gravity reading for each 3 C that the urine temperature is above the calibration temperature of the urinometer, and subtract 0.001 for each 3 C that it is below the calibration temperature.

2. pH

Dip a short strip of Nitrazine® paper into the urine, shake off any excess urine and compare the wet paper with the color chart to find the pH between 4.5 and 7.5 pH units to nearest 0.5 unit. Subtract 0.2 from the indicated pH value on the chart for the actual urine pH.

3. Protein

a. Sulfosalicylic Acid Test*
1. Dissolve 200 g sodium sulfate by heating in 750 ml water. Cool; add 50 g sulfosalicylic acid, and dilute to 1 liter with water.
2. Mix equal parts of filtered urine or the supernatant of centrifuged urine and this sulfosalicylic acid reagent in a test tube.
3. Grade the degree of cloudiness as the tube is held against a dark background.
4. Figure 23 on page 160 shows the results of the Sulfosalicylic Acid Test done on four urine samples. From left to right, the grading of the proteinuria and the actual amount of protein (albumin) pres-

---

*Note that cephalosporin antibiotics give a precipitate with sulfosalicylic acid.

ent are: 1+ (30 mg/100 ml urine), 2+ (100 mg/100 ml urine), 3+ (300 mg/100 ml urine) and 4+ (1000 mg/100 ml urine).

b. Reagent Strip Test (Albustix®)
Dip a commercially prepared reagent impregnated paper stick (Albustix®) into the urine and match against color standards.

4. Bence Jones Protein

Add 3 percent acetic acid drop by drop to 10 ml of urine in a test tube to bring the pH to 5.0 as measured with Nitrazine® paper. Bring the mixture to a boil. Filter it through a hot funnel to remove any heat-precipitated ordinary protein. Using a thermometer, observe to see the appearance of a cloud of Bence Jones protein between 70 C and 45 C as the urine cools. This dissolves on cooling below 45 C.

5. Blood

a. Reagent Strip Test (Hemastix®)
Dip a prepared paper stick (Hemastix®) into the urine and compare the color with a color chart at one minute.

6. Glucose

a. Glucose Oxidase Tests
Dip paper strips (Tes-Tape®) or sticks (Clinistix®) impregnated with glucose oxidase enzyme into the urine and match against color standards according to the directions. These tests are specific for D-glucose.

b. Reagent Tablet Test (Clinitest®)
Put five drops of urine and ten drops of water in a test tube. Drop one Clinitest® tablet into the test tube. Do not shake the test tube during the reaction, nor for 15 seconds after boiling has stopped. Fifteen seconds after boiling stops shake the test tube gently and compare the color of the solution with the color chart. All shades of blue are negative. Ignore the whitish sediment. Color changes that develop after the 15-second waiting period should be disregarded. This test also gives a positive reaction with reducing sugars other than glucose and with other reducing substances.

7. Ketone Bodies

Acetone and Acetoacetic Acid
1. Reagent Tablet Test (Acetest®): Put on a commercially prepared tablet (Acetest®) one drop of urine. Compare the color at 30 seconds with a color chart.

2. Reagent Strip Test (Ketostix®): Commercially prepared paper sticks (Ketostix®) are dipped in the urine and compared after 15 seconds with a color chart.

8. Phenylpyruvic Acid

Reagent Strip Test (Phenistix®)
Reagent strips (Phenistix®) are dipped in urine and compared with a color chart at one-half minute. (Salicylates and phenothiazines give a pink to brownish purple color.)

9. Bilirubin

a. Foam Test
Shake the tube or jug containing the urine. Look for a yellow color of the *foam*. Protein in the urine gives an increased amount of white foam.

b. Reagent Tablet Test (Ictotest®)
Place five drops of urine on one square of special test mat. Place a reagent tablet in the center of this moistened area. Cover the tablet with two drops of water. With a positive test for bilirubin a blue or purple color forms on the test mat around the reagent tablet within 30 seconds. The test is negative for bilirubin when no blue or purple color forms within 30 seconds around the reagent tablet. The sensitivity of this test permits detection of 0.1 to 0.05 mg bilirubin per 100 ml urine.

E. Stains For Bacteriologic Examination of the Urine

1. Methylene Blue Stain

Loffler's alkaline methylene blue stain is composed of 30 parts of a saturated alcoholic solution of methylene blue and 100 parts of a 1:10,000 aqueous solution of potassium hydroxide. It is applied for one-half to three minutes to a dried centrifuged urine sediment that has been spread on a slide and fixed by passage through a flame. The stain is then rinsed off with water. After drying, the slide may be examined microscopically using the oil immersion lens. This simple stain for detecting the presence of bacteriuria is easy to use.

2. Gram Stain

Allow the centrifuged urine sediment that has been spread on a slide to dry. Fix it by passage through a flame. Cover the slide with a solution of 2 g crystal violet in 100 ml methyl alcohol. Allow it to stand for one minute; then wash. Cover the slide with Gram's iodine solution for one minute. (Gram's iodine solution is composed of iodine 1.0 g, potassium iodide 2.0 g, and distilled water 300 ml.) Wash off the Gram's iodine, then decolorize for approximately 30 seconds by flooding the slide with 95 percent alcohol. Counterstain for 15 to 20 seconds by covering the slide with a 1 percent aqueous solution of safranin. Wash the slide with water, then dry. This is a more difficult stain to use; however, it yields more information about the type of bacteria present than does the methylene blue stain. For example, knowing that a Gram-negative bacillus or a Gram-positive coccus is the predominant organism, permits more rational therapy of the urinary tract infection to be instituted pending definitive identification of the organism by culture.

3. Ziehl-Neelsen Stain

Prepare the slide of the urine sediment as above, but the sediment should be derived from a 24-hour urine collection. Flood the slide with carbol fuchsin* and heat it gently until it steams for five minutes. Wash it with water, then decolorize with acid alcohol for one-half to two minutes. Wash with water, then counterstain with methylene blue stain for one minute. Examine the dry slide with the oil immersion lens of the microscope. Use this stain when tuberculosis of the urinary tract is suspected. It provides a means for rapidly determining the presence of acid-fast organisms. Failure to see acid-fast organisms does not mean that they are absent, of

*Dilute 10 ml of a saturated solution of basic fuchsin in ethyl alcohol with 90 ml of a 5 percent aqueous solution of phenol.

course. Culture and guinea-pig innoculation of the sediment should also always be done for positive identification of the *tubercle bacillus* and assessment of its pathogenicity.

F. Methods for Evaluating Kidney Function

1. Fishberg Concentration Test

Allow the patient to ingest no fluids from 8 PM until 10 AM the next day. The evening meal must contain less than 200 ml of total fluid. Discard any night urine. Collect the specimens voided on arising, at 8 AM and at 10 AM. Determine the specific gravity of each. In normal individuals one or more of the urine specimens will have a specific gravity of 1.023 or higher. *Note:* Performance of this test may be dangerous for patients having renal insufficiency.

2. Fifteen-Minute PSP Test

Have the patient drink 600 ml water. When the patient feels some urge to urinate, inject intravenously exactly 1 ml phenolsulfonphthalein solution (6 mg). Note the exact time of the injection. Collect all of the urine that the patient can void at *exactly* 15 minutes after the injection. Add a few ml of 10 percent sodium hydroxide solution (sufficient to make it alkaline) to the urine specimen and dilute the entire specimen to 1 liter in a graduated cylinder with distilled water.

Compare a test tube full of the diluted specimen with color standards to determine the percent of the injected dye excreted. The lower limit for the normal excretion of the dye is 23 percent in 15 minutes. Most normal individuals will excrete more than 30 percent.

3. Twenty-four-Hour Creatinine Clearance

An accurately timed 24-hour urine is collected and its total volume is measured. A blood sample for determination of the serum creatinine is obtained. The creatinine concentrations determined in both serum and urine are used in the following calculation:

$$C_{creatinine} = \frac{UV}{P}$$

where U = urine creatinine concentration in g per liter
V = 24-hour urine volume in liters
P = serum creatinine concentration in mg per 100 ml divided by 100

The normal 24-hour creatinine clearance is 170 liters per 1.73 m^2 body surface area.

atlas of
urine sediments

atlas of
urine sediments

A. Black-and-White Figures

B. Color Figures

FIGURE NO.	CONTENTS OF FIGURES
11	Oil immersion view of a stained urine sediment. Cell **A** is a Sternheimer-Malbin positive poly. Note its swollen cytoplasm. Cell **B** is a renal tubular epithelial cell. Note the squamous epithelial cell in the left-lower corner.
12	A high-power view of a stained urine sediment showing squamous epithelial cells (**A**), Sternheimer-Malbin positive polys (**B** and **D**), red blood cells (**C**), and a coarsely granular cast just above the letter **B**. Note that it has parallel sides.
13	The large object in this high-power magnification of an unstained urine sediment is a hyaline cast. It does have a few small inclusions. The larger cell below the cast contains refractile fatty material. Most of the other cells are red blood cells.
14	Low-power view of an unstained urine sediment viewed with too much light.
15	The same urine sediment shown in the previous figure is viewed with reduced illumination. One can now see a predominantly hyaline cast and a red blood cell (**A**).
16	Low-power view of a stained urine sediment showing a a squamous epithelial cell (**A**) and hyaline casts, such as **B** and **C**.
17	A high-power view of a stained urine sediment. Extending into the right upper quadrant of the figure is a cellular cast. This cast contains polys, such as cell **B**. Red blood cells are also present (**A**).
18	Low-power, stained view of a hyaline cast.
19	A high-power view of an unstained urine sediment showing red blood cells (**A** and **B**), red blood cell cast (between letters **C** and **D**), and renal tubular epithelial cells or polys (like **C** and **D**). (In the unstained preparation it is hard to distinguish one from the other.) Just above the middle of line **D** there is an oval fat body.
20	A high-power view of a stained urine sediment containing red blood cells (**A** and **D**), renal tubular epithelial cells (**B**), and a renal tubular epithelial cell cast (**C**).
21	An oil immersion view of a stained renal tubular epithelial cell cast.

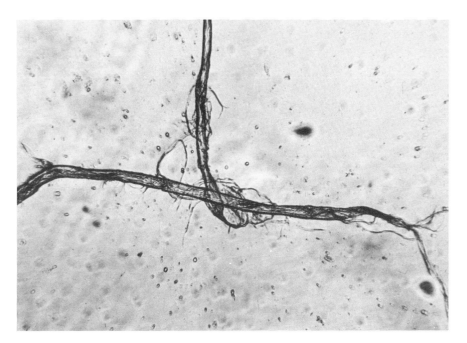

Figure 1

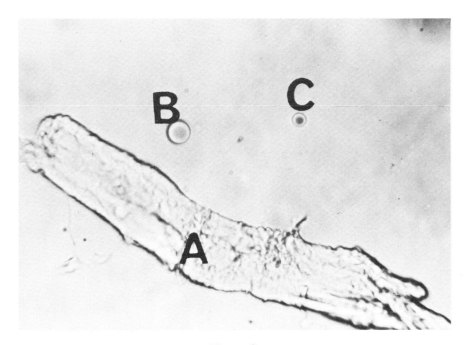

Figure 2

Figure 3

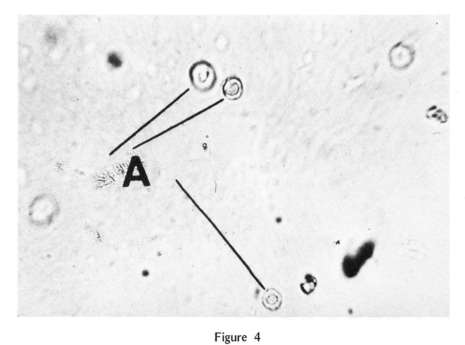

Figure 4

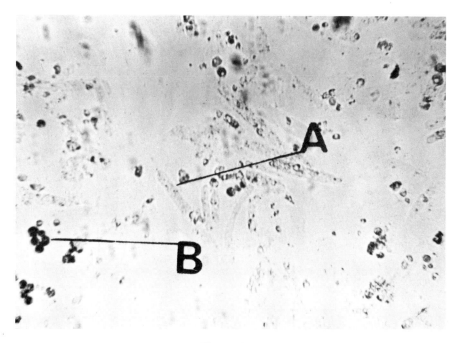

Figure 5

Figure 6

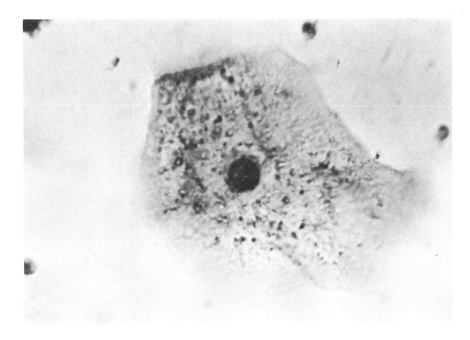

Figure 7

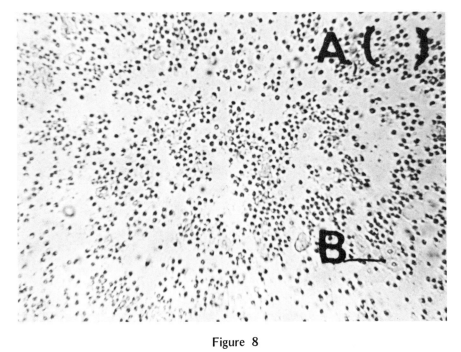

Figure 8

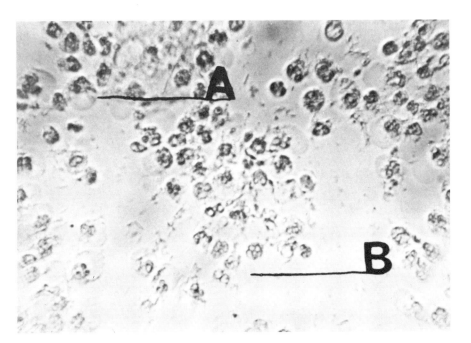

Figure 9

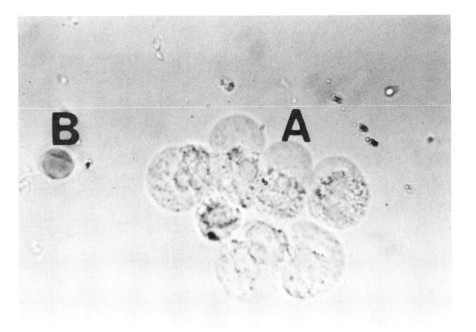

Figure 10

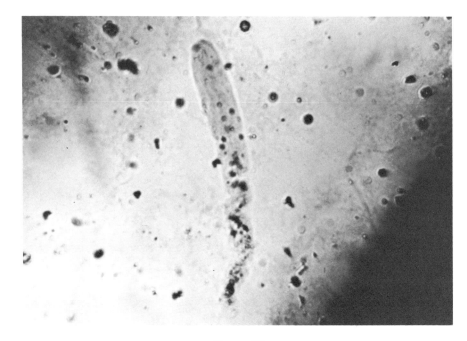

Figure 11

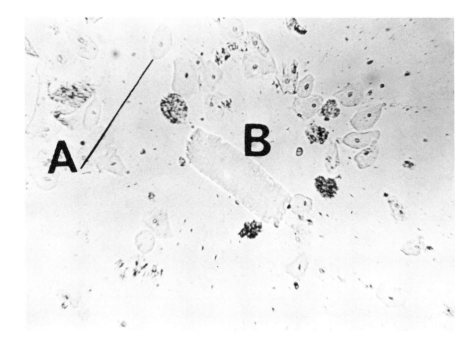

Figure 12

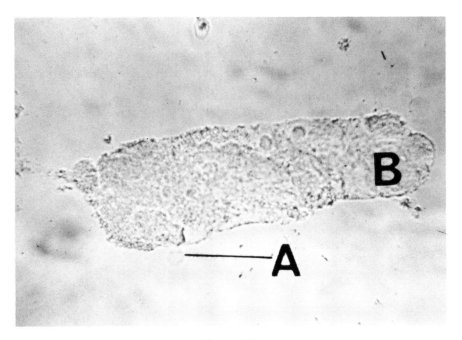

Figure 13

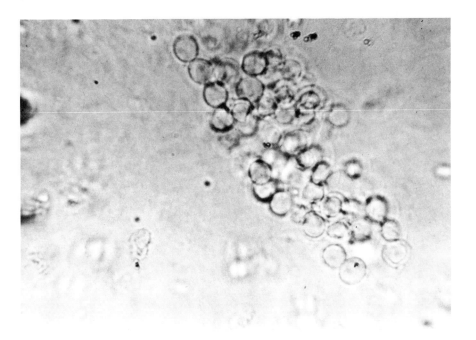

Figure 14

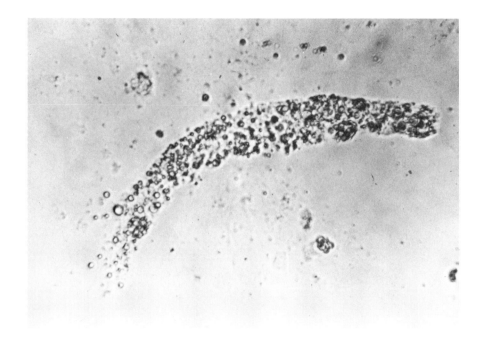

Figure 15

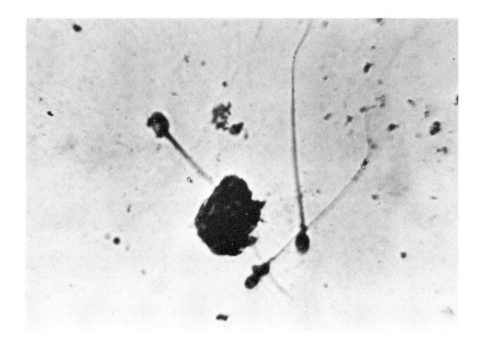

Figure 16

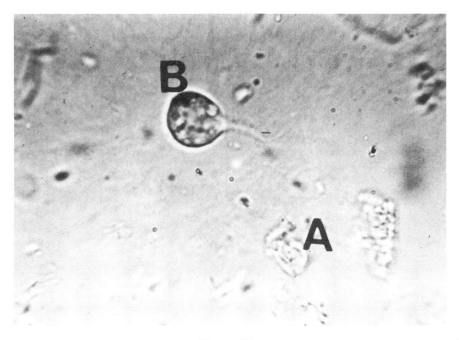

Figure 17

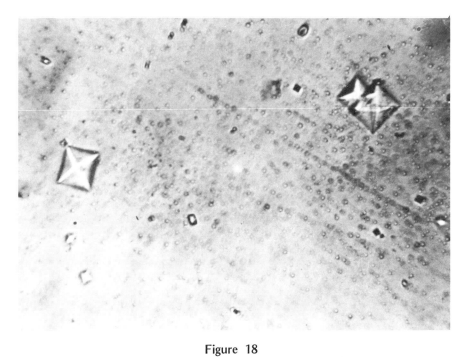

Figure 18

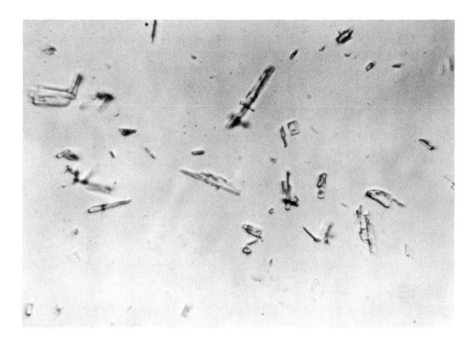

Figure 19

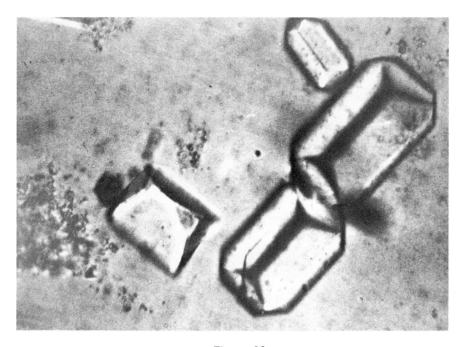

Figure 20

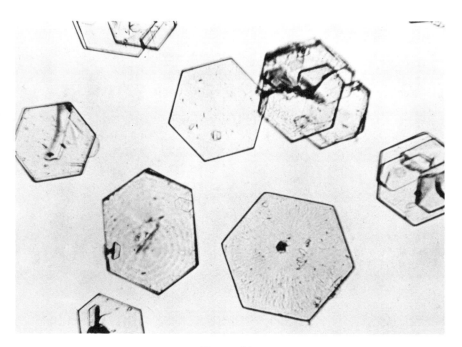

Figure 21

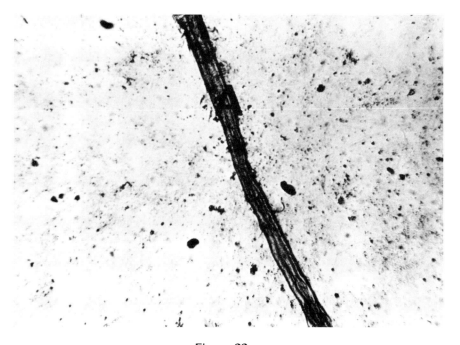

Figure 22

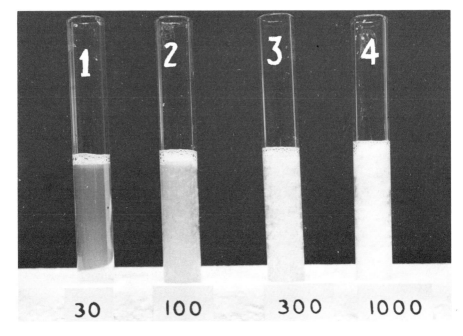

Figure 23

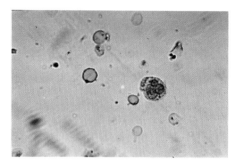

Figure 1

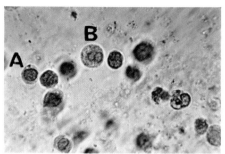

Figure 2

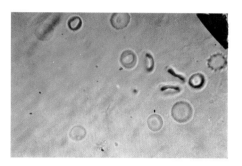

Figure 3

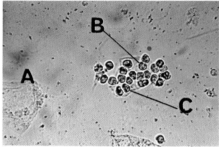

Figure 4

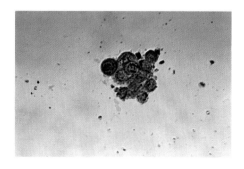

Figure 5

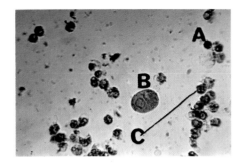

Figure 6

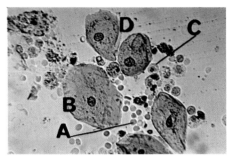

Figure 7

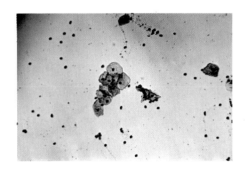

Figure 8

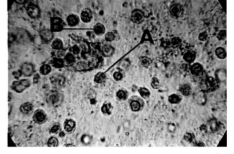

Figure 9

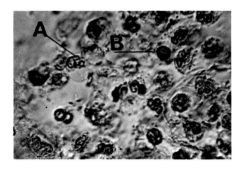

Figure 10

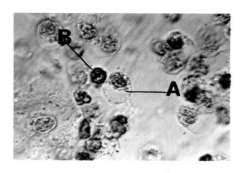

Figure 11

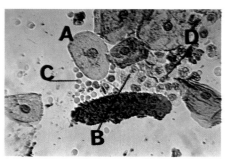

Figure 12

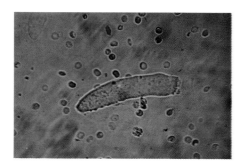

Figure 13

Figure 14

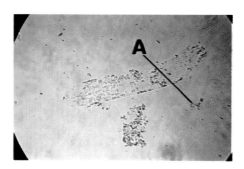

Figure 15

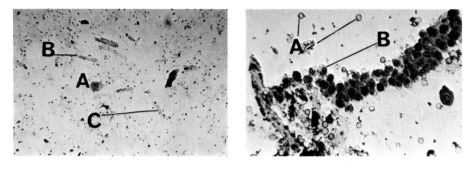

Figure 16   Figure 17

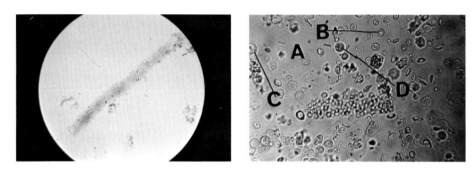

Figure 18   Figure 19

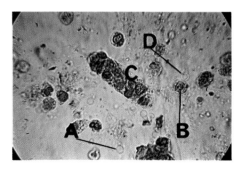

Figure 20

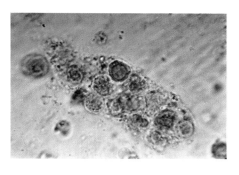

Figure 21

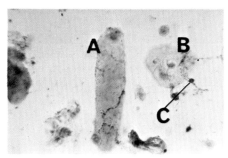

Figure 22

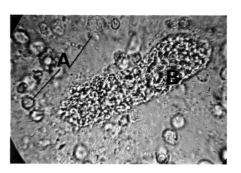

Figure 23

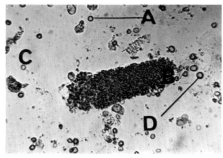

Figure 24

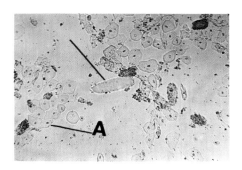

Figure 25

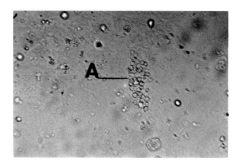

Figure 26

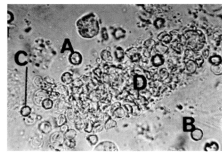

Figure 27

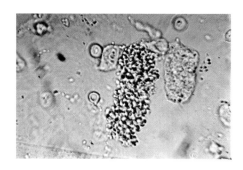

Figure 28

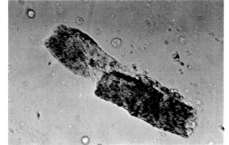

Figure 29

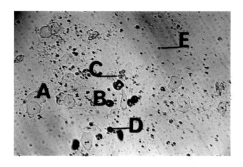

Figure 30

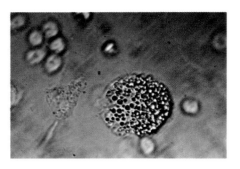

Figure 31

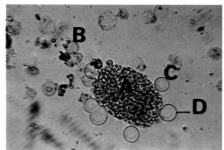

Figure 32

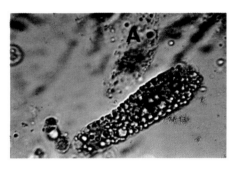

Figure 33

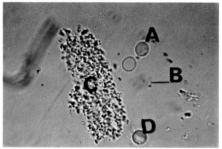

Figure 34

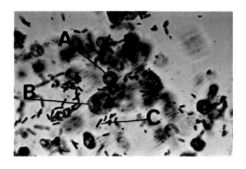

Figure 35

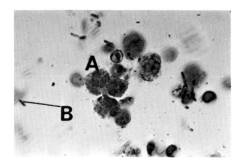

Figure 36

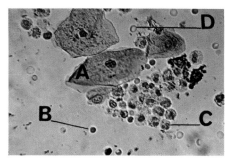

Figure 37

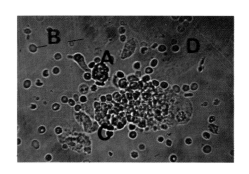

Figure 38

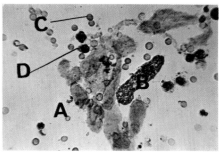

Figure 39

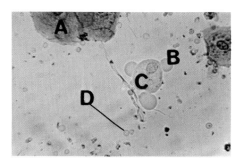

Figure 40